Imaging of
Vertebral Trauma

CLINICAL DIAGNOSTIC IMAGING SERIES
Morrie E. Kricun, Series Editor
Associate Professor
Department of Radiology
Musculoskeletal Section
Hospital of the University of Pennsylvania
Philadelphia, Pennsylvania

Imaging of Vertebral Trauma
Richard H. Daffner

Imaging of the Foot and Ankle
D. M. Forrester, Morrie E. Kricun, and Roger Kerr

Imaging of the Pelvis
Madeleine R. Fisher and Morrie E. Kricun

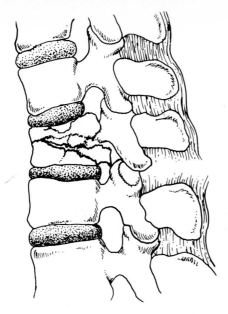

Morrie E. Kricun, Series Editor

Imaging of
Vertebral Trauma

Richard H. Daffner, M.D.
Clinical Professor of Radiology
University of Pittsburgh School of Medicine
and
Department of Diagnostic Radiology
Allegheny General Hospital
Pittsburgh, Pennsylvania

AN ASPEN PUBLICATION®
Aspen Publishers, Inc.
Rockville, Maryland
Royal Tunbridge Wells
1988

Library of Congress Cataloging-in-Publication Data

Daffner, Richard H., 1941- .
Imaging of vertebral trauma/Richard H. Daffner.

"An Aspen publication."
Includes bibliographies and index.
ISBN: 0-87189-767-9
1. Vertebrae--Wounds and injuries--Diagnosis--Atlases.
2. Vertebrae-Imaging--Atlases. I. Title. II. Series.
[DNLM: 1. Spinal Injuries--radiography--atlases. WE 17 D124]
RD533.D24   1988   617'.3750757--dc19
DNLM/DLC
for Library of Congress
88-6329
CIP

The authors have made every effort to ensure the accuracy of the information herein,
particularly with regard to drug selection and dose. However, appropriate information
sources should be consulted, especially for new or unfamiliar drugs or procedures. It is
the responsibility of every practitioner to evaluate the appropriateness of a particular
opinion in the context of actual clinical situations and with due consideration to new
developments. Authors, editors, and the publisher cannot be held responsible for any
typographical or other errors found in this book.

Editorial Services: Ruth Bloom

Library of Congress Catalog Card Number: 88-6329
ISBN: 0-87189-767-9

Printed in the United States of America

1 2 3 4 5

To
William F. Barry, Jr. (Deceased)
George J. Baylin
and
John A. Gehweiler, Jr.

Teachers, scholars, friends

Table of Contents

Foreword

The recent advances in technology in the field of medical imaging have greatly facilitated the initial evaluation and follow-up care of patients who sustain spinal trauma. The rising interest in traumatology, coupled with the need to image the traumatized spine, has created a need for a reference on imaging modalities available for the evaluation of spinal trauma victims.

Imaging of Vertebral Trauma, written by Richard H. Daffner, MD, is an outstanding book that deals with the state of the art in imaging of the traumatized spine. It is well written, concise, easy to read, and well illustrated. Dr. Daffner, an authority in the field of imaging of spinal trauma, shares his vast experience with illustrative cases, pertinent discussions, informative tables, and up-to-date references. In his discussions, Dr. Daffner has placed the various imaging modalities in a proper perspective regarding the work-up of the patient. He appropriately stresses the importance of the conventional radiograph by explaining in an analytical way the approach to the radiographic evaluation, the analysis of the radiographic signs of spinal injury, and the correlation of the radiographic signs of the underlying mechanisms of injury. The other modalities are used to complement the discussions of the various types of injuries.

Chapter 1 defines the descriptive terms of fractures and dislocations, discusses the terminology used in reporting traumatic abnormalities, and defines the basic mechanisms of injury. Chapter 2 presents basic practical anatomy of the spine and sacrum using line drawings, conventional radiographs, and radiographs of anatomic specimens. Chapter 3 presents a more in-depth discussion of the modalities available for imaging the traumatized spine, including conventional radiography, conventional polydirectional tomography, computed tomography, magnetic resonance imaging, and myelography. The advantages, limitations, indications, technical considerations, and comparison with other modalities are discussed. Chapter 4 covers the mechanisms of injury and what the author calls the "Fingerprints" of injury, namely the patterns of radiographic signs that identify the underlying mechanism of injury. Chapter 5 presents the "ABCS" of radiographic interpretations, an analytical approach to the evaluation of the conventional radiograph. In addition, there is a discussion of radiographic and computed tomographic findings of vertebral injuries. Normal variants that may mimic fractures and pseudofractures are discussed in Chapter 6.

Dr. Daffner has succeeded in his goals. He has provided a book that represents a practical and systematic approach to the understanding of the radiographic signs of spinal trauma and their underlying mechanism of injury. He has provided an appreciation and understanding of the importance, use, and interpretation of the newer imaging modalities such as computed tomography and magnetic resonance imaging. I am very pleased to have been able to write the foreword to this important and immensely helpful book.

Morrie E. Kricun, MD
June 1988

Preface

Vertebral trauma is a major cause of permanent disability. Although there has been an increasing number of vertebral injuries due to motor vehicle accidents, improved medical technology has salvaged the lives of individuals who suffer what were once considered uniformly fatal injuries. The key to the administration of prompt therapy and rehabilitation is the ability to properly diagnose the full extent of these injuries. The discovery of the roentgen ray was the first major technological breakthrough in diagnosing vertebral trauma, and this method remained the chief method for diagnosis until the development of computed tomography and magnetic resonance imaging. With these methods it is now possible to define the full extent of injury and, in the latter method, to determine the extent of spinal cord involvement.

I became interested in the subject of vertebral injury through my long and close association with Dr John A Gehweiler, who described many signs of subtle injury to the cervical vertebrae. The advent of multiplanar imaging confirmed the validity of the signs described by Dr Gehweiler and other individuals in-terested in vertebral trauma. This book grew out of a series of lectures that I have given over the past decade and represents a systematic and practical approach to the radiography of vertebral trauma. This book is not encyclopedic in scope and does not describe every variation of every type of vertebral injury. It does, however, provide a working basis for the practicing radiologist in the community hospital as well as in the large medical center, who is often the first person called on to interpret radiographs of a patient with vertebral injury. The book relies on the premise that all injuries (vertebral and nonvertebral) occur in a predictable and reproducible fashion that is solely dependent on the mechanism of injury. As such, each type of injury produces indelible signs that I have termed ''fingerprints.'' By following this logical approach and by applying the principles outlined in the text, the reader will gain confidence in his or her diagnostic skills and ability to diagnose even the most subtle injury.

Richard H. Daffner, MD

Acknowledgments

No book of this scope could be produced without the technical assistance of many individuals. I am extremely grateful to Ms Maggie Cauley for her long hours in manuscript preparation, editing, and collation. I am also indebted to Mr Gary Stark of the Creative Services Department at Allegheny General Hospital and to other members of the staff, including Ms Mary Jane Bent, Mr Bill Brattina, Mr Paul Jorgensen, Ms Donna Spillane, Mr Frank Stinelli, and Mr Doug Whitman for production of the illustrations. In particular, I wish to thank Mr Scott Williams for the superb artwork; I also acknowledge the artwork of Ms Debbie Whitman and Mr Maurice Williams. For their assistance in clinical correlation of the case material in the book, I also wish to thank Daniel L Diamond, MD, head of the Trauma Center at Allegheny General Hospital; Joseph C Maroon, MD, head of the Department of Neurosurgery, and his colleagues; Parviz Baghai, MD; James E Wilberger, MD; E Richard Prostko, MD; and Randall L Sherman, MD. Finally, I thank Ms Susan Sherwin for miscellaneous secretarial assistance, and my dear wife Alva for her encouragement, support, and patience as well as her editorial skills in proofreading and editing the manuscript and galleys.

Richard H. Daffner, MD

Chapter 1

An Overview of the Radiologic Diagnosis of Vertebral Injuries

In the history of humankind, no injury has evoked greater fear than vertebral fracture or dislocation. These injuries are among the most devastating and result in a gamut of abnormalities that rank from mild pain and discomfort to severe paralysis and even death. Despite improved technology for the diagnosis and treatment of these injuries, the physician who is confronted with a ''spine-injured patient'' often feels incapable of interpreting radiographic studies that would delineate the full extent of injury.

This book presents a systematic approach to the diagnosis of vertebral trauma that the author has used for the interpretation of radiographs of patients with vertebral injury. Furthermore, it amplifies several concepts that the author has developed, namely, that vertebral injuries occur in a predictable pattern, that the radiographic changes produced by a generic injury are similar, and that the findings for injuries due to the same mechanism are identical no matter where they are encountered within the vertebral column.[7]

This chapter defines the descriptive terms regarding fractures and dislocations, reviews the terminology used for reporting these abnormalities, and discusses basic mechanisms of injury. Succeeding chapters discuss anatomy, imaging methods available for diagnosing vertebral injuries, and the basic diagnostic principles that make possible a logical and systematic approach to vertebral injuries. The final chapter discusses normal variants and pseudofractures.

FRACTURES

Most medical dictionaries define a fracture as a disruption, either complete or incomplete, in the continuity of a bone, epiphyseal plate, or cartilaginous joint surface. The author prefers a different definition that has more practical significance. According to this definition, a fracture is a soft tissue injury in which a bone is broken. This definition is of greatest importance in injuries to the skull and to the vertebral column, where the bony disruption itself may be the least important component of the injury and damage to the meninges, brain, spinal cord, or peripheral nerves is more serious.

There are a number of descriptive terms that are used in regard to fractures. Most of these are applicable to the peripheral skeleton. A complete fracture is one in which both cortexes of a bone have been broken; an incomplete fracture involves only one cortex. In closed or simple fractures, there is no communication of the fracture site with the exterior of the body; in open or compound fractures, there is communication between the fracture site and the external environment. Most fractures of the vertebral column are closed. Open fractures generally result from missile injuries. Operative intervention converts a closed fracture to an open one.

Fractures may be the result of either direct or indirect injury. In a direct injury, force is applied directly to the bone and fracture occurs at the site of impact. In the vertebral column,

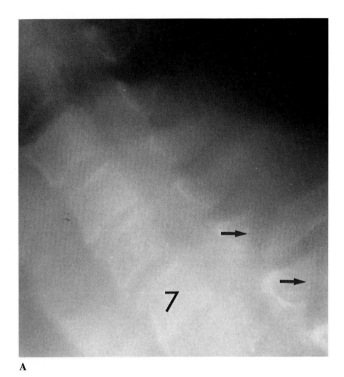

A

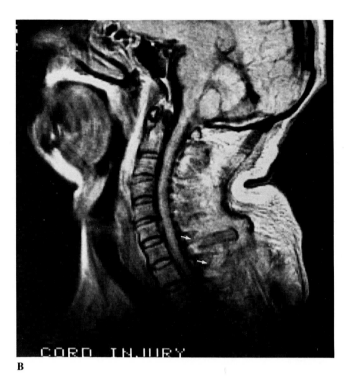

B

Figure 1-1 "Clay-shoveler" fracture of C-7. The patient was struck with a baseball bat during an altercation. **(A)** Lateral tomogram shows fractures of spinous processes of C-7 and T-1 (arrows). **(B)** Sagittal magnetic resonance imaging (MRI) examination (T_R = 2.1, T_E = 90) shows similar findings (arrows).

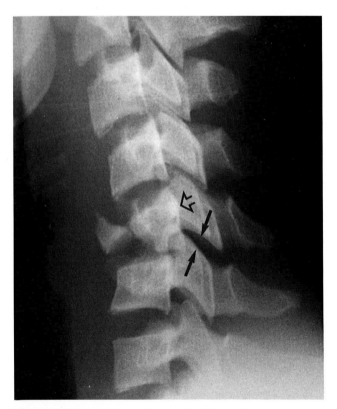

Figure 1-2 "Teardrop" burst fracture of C-5 in a patient who dove into shallow water. The vertical axial force resulted in bursting of C-5 with retropulsion of a fragment of bone (open arrow), retrolisthesis, and widening of the facet joints (thin arrows).

this is most likely to occur in a spinous process (Fig 1-1).[5] The vast majority of vertebral injuries result from indirect trauma, in which force is applied at a distance from the involved vertebra (Fig 1-2). In the case of cervical injury, a loading force applied to the head or trunk is transmitted directly to the vertebral column, resulting in a deformity far beyond the normal physiologic range of motion. Sudden acceleration or deceleration of the head relative to the trunk, or vice versa (as often occurs in traffic accidents), will also produce indirect injury, particularly in the cervical region.[1–4,6–14]

JOINT INJURIES

Joint injuries result from the same types of forces that produce fractures. The mildest form of joint injury is a ligamentous sprain due to stretching of ligamentous fibers beyond their normal range of elasticity. This results in small tears and hemorrhages. Rupture of a ligament may occur with more severe injury. The only difference between a sprain and a rupture is the degree of injury.

Sprain or rupture of a ligament or a combination of ligaments may result in three types of joint instability: occult, luxation, and dislocation. Occult instability may be recognized radiographically only when a joint is stressed (Fig 1-3). Luxation is a more severe joint injury in which there is partial loss of contact between apposing joint surfaces (Fig 1-4). Dislocation is complete loss of contact between apposing articular surfaces (Fig 1-5). The term locking refers to an abnormal

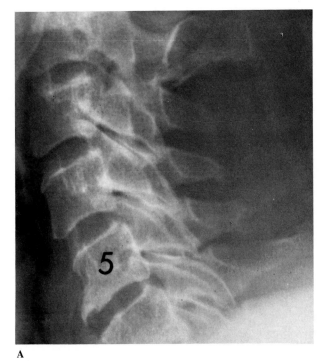

A

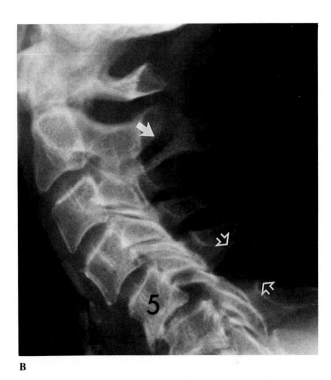

B

Figure 1-3 Occult instability: flexion sprain of C-5 in a 72-year-old woman involved in a rear-end automobile accident. (**A**) Supine radiograph shows mild degenerative changes. (**B**) Upright radiograph shows anterolisthesis of C-5 on C-6, narrowing of the C-5 disk space, widening of the interspinous spaces (open arrows), and fracture through the spinous process of C-2 (closed arrow). There has been nearly complete loss of continuity along the articular surfaces of the facet joints of C-5 and C-6. This case illustrates the need for erect radiographs before a patient is discharged from the hospital.

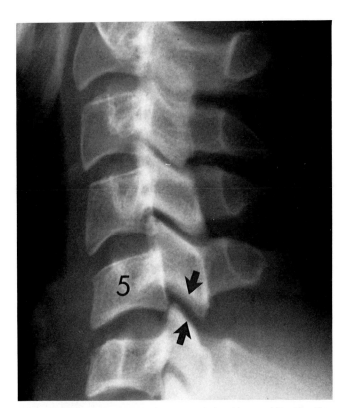

Figure 1-4 Luxation instability: flexion sprain in a 22-year-old involved in a motor vehicle accident. There is kyphotic angulation at C-5, widening of the interspinous space at C-5, and widening of the facet joint of C5-6 with partial loss of contact (arrows).

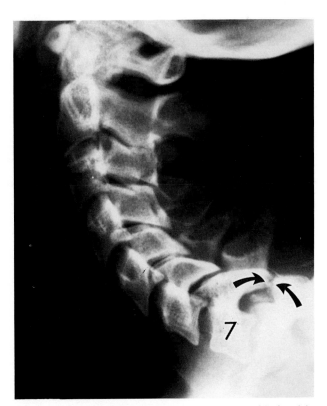

Figure 1-5 Cervical dislocation of C-7 and T-1 with locking of the facet joints (arrows). There is complete loss of continuity of the bony surfaces. The patient was neurologically intact.

relationship that results from dislocation between articular surfaces (Fig 1-6).

DESCRIPTIVE TERMINOLOGY

Fractures and dislocations in the axial skeleton are described by the same terms as those in the peripheral skeleton. By convention, an injury should be defined at the level or levels at which it has occurred. When an injury occurs at a disk level, it is defined by the vertebra above it. Thus an injury to the C4-5 disk space is said to have occurred at the C-4 disk space.

Descriptive terms such as avulsion, impaction, distraction, rotation, compression, and burst should all be used. The plane of fracture (horizontal, transverse, coronal, or sagittal) and displacement of major fragments should also be described. In addition, if a fracture appears to be due to a pathologic etiology, this should be stated. Figures 1-7 through 1-11 show examples of various fractures and the descriptive terminology to be used for these injuries.

Joint injuries are always described by relating the direction taken by the upper vertebra with regard to the one below. This is in contradistinction to the descriptive terminology used for peripheral fractures, where the position and angulation of the distal fragment are described in relation to the proximal frag-

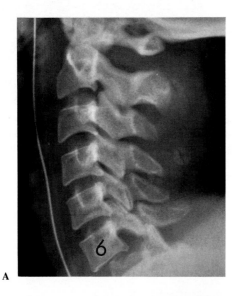

A

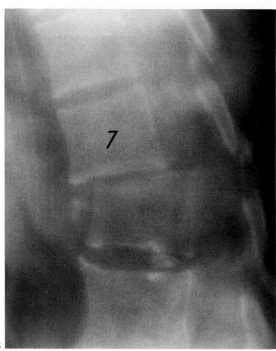

B

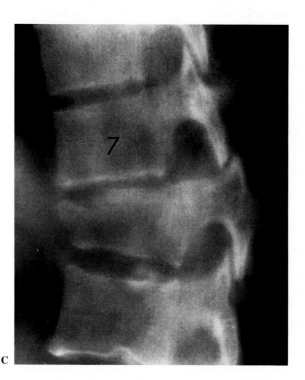

C

Figure 1-6 Dislocation with locking of facet joints. **(A)** Cervical dislocation of C-6 on C-7 with bilateral facet locking. **(B and C)** Thoracic fracture dislocation of T-7 on T-8. Tomograms show the locked facets.

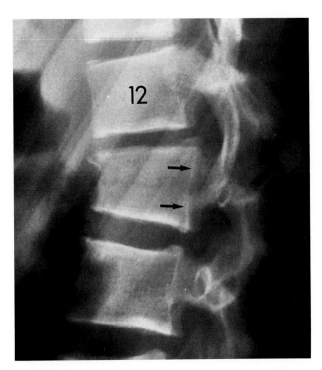

Figure 1-7 Simple flexion injury of L-1. There is loss of height at the anterior portion of the body of L-1, and the T-12 disk space is narrowed. The posterior vertebral body line of L-1 (arrows) is intact. Compare with Fig. 1-8, a burst fracture.

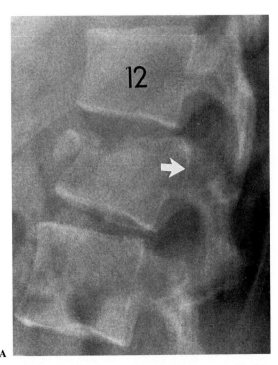

A

Figure 1-8 Burst fracture of L-1 in an unrestrained automobile driver who was thrown from the vehicle. The patient was paraplegic. **(A)** A lateral radiograph shows compression of the body of L-1 and comminution. There is retropulsion of a fragment of bone from the posterior vertebral body line (arrow) to encroach on the vertebral canal. In addition, there is anterior wedging of the body of T-12. Compare with Figure 1-7.

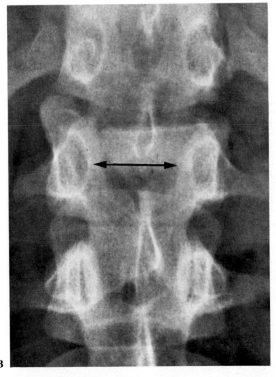

B

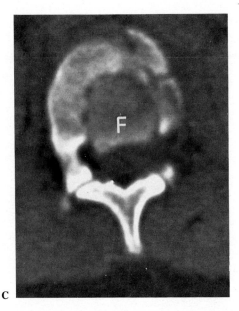

C

Figure 1-8 (B) Frontal view shows loss of height of L-1, comminution, and widening of the interpedicular distance (arrows). **(C)** CT scan shows comminution of the body of L-1 with retropulsion of a central fragment (F) to encroach on the vertebral canal.

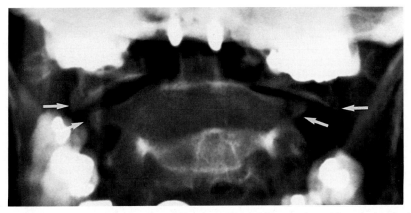
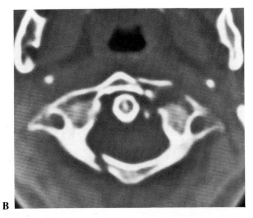

Figure 1-9 Jefferson fracture of C-1. **(A)** Open-mouth frontal radiograph shows bilateral atlanto-axial dissociation (arrows). **(B)** CT scan shows the fractures through the anterior and posterior arches of C-1.

ment. Figures 1-12 through 1-14 show variations of joint injuries and their descriptive terminologies.

A number of terms are used throughout this book in regard to the mechanisms of injury.[2,5–9,13,14] Although these terms are defined in further detail in Chapter 4, they require a brief description at this time.

Flexion injuries result from a forward bending motion of the vertebral column at any level. This may be the result of posterior impact of an indirect force on the vertebral column or anterior impact of the torso on a solid object.[6,14] Similarly,

extension injuries are due to a posterior bending of the vertebral column in response to either an anterior force or sudden deceleration against a solid object posteriorly.[7,12,13]

Shearing injuries are the result of horizontally oriented forces being transmitted to the vertebral column from any direction. The normal vertebral column is permitted limited motion in flexion and extension and even more limited motion in rotation. Horizontal motion is never normal.[7]

Rotational injuries result from abnormal torque applied to the vertebral column. Again, very limited rotation is possible

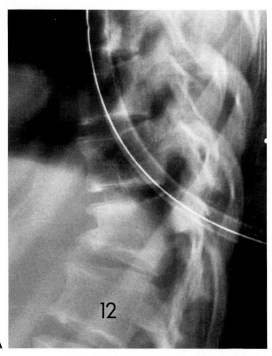
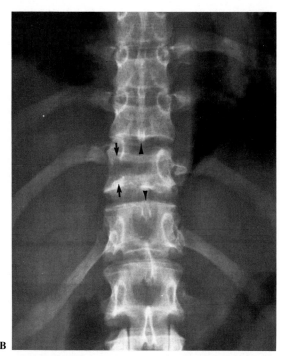

Figure 1-10 Smith-type fracture of T-11. The patient, involved in an automobile accident, was wearing a lap-type seatbelt. **(A)** Lateral film shows lateral compression of T-11 anteriorly and posterior distraction. **(B)** Frontal view shows that T-11 has literally been torn in two along the horizontal plane. Note the fracture of the pedicle on the right (arrows) and widening of the interspinous space (arrowheads).

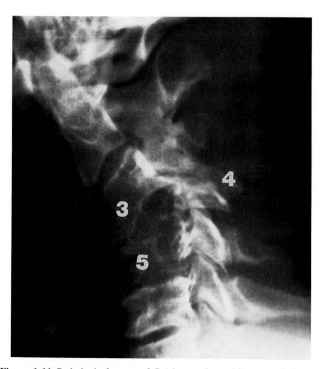

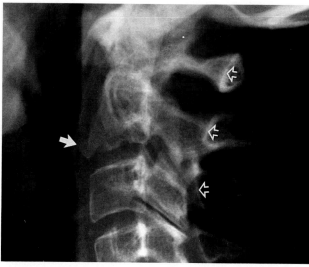

Figure 1-12 Extension injury of C-2. Lateral radiographs show a fracture of the anterior-inferior portion of the body of C-2 (solid arrow). There is slight retrolisthesis of C-2 on C-3 as evidenced by disruption of the spinolaminar line (open arrows).

Figure 1-11 Pathologic fracture of C-4 in a patient with metastatic breast carcinoma. The body of C-4 has been almost completely destroyed. There is forward collapse of C-3 on C-5 and metastatic lesions in C-2, C-3, and C-5.

only in the upper cervical region. Rotary injuries to the thoracolumbar area usually result in severe neurologic compromise because they are extremely disruptive.[7]

All the above mechanisms may occur in combination. In addition, they take into account the effect of axial loading.

ETIOLOGY OF VERTEBRAL INJURIES

The vast majority of vertebral injuries are due to motor vehicle accidents. This accounts for 85% of the patients seen at our institution's trauma center. In almost all these cases there were three coincident events: speed, greater than 15 miles per hour over the posted limit; alcohol, greater than 0.1 mg % (the legal limit in most states); and total lack of use of seatbelts. In a recent review of nearly 1000 patients with vertebral injuries due to automobile accidents, only 10 patients were wearing seatbelts at the time of injury. In all the other patients, the vast majority of lesions could have been prevented by use of a seatbelt.[7]

In a study of vertebral trauma patients at our institution, approximately 14% of injuries resulted from falls. This is the second most common etiology of vertebral injury. Miscellaneous causes, such as diving accidents and missile injuries, accounted for the remaining 1% of injuries seen in this study.[7]

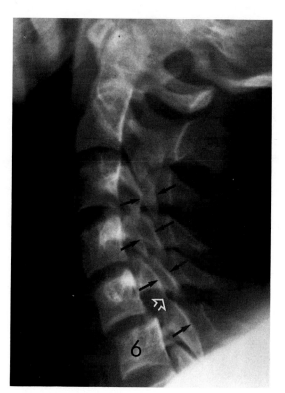

Figure 1-13 Unilateral facet lock of C-5 on C-6. Lateral radiograph shows a single facet shadow at C-6 and a duplicated facet shadow (arrows) above, indicating rotation of the vertebrae above C-6. The open arrow indicates the point of locking.

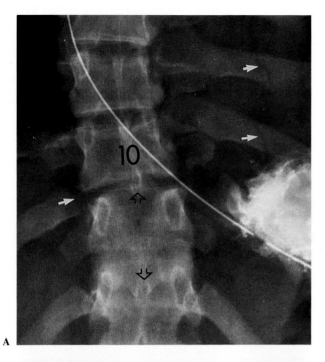

A

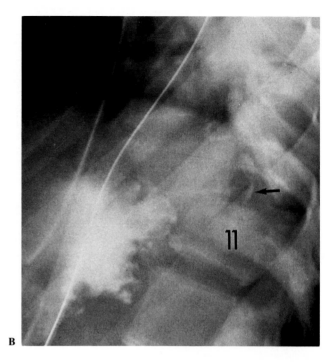

B

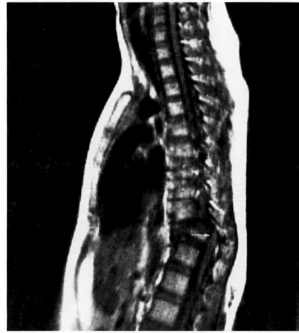

C

Figure 1-14 Dislocation of T-10 on T-11. **(A)** Frontal radiographs of an unrestrained front-seat passenger who was thrown from the vehicle. There is laterolisthesis of T-10 on T-11 to the right. In addition, there is widening of the interspinous space between T-10 and T-11 (open arrows) and multiple rib fractures (solid arrows). This radiograph does not convey the full extent of damage. **(B)** Lateral radiograph shows third-degree spondylolisthesis of T-10 on T-11. A small fragment of bone from the posterior lip of T-10 is visible (arrow). **(C)** MRI study ($T_R = 0.3$, $T_E = 15$) shows the extent of damage, including spinal cord transection (arrow).

REFERENCES

1. Alker GJ Jr, Oh YS, Leslie EV, et al: Postmortem radiology of head and neck injuries in fatal traffic accidents. *Radiology* 1975;114:611–617.

2. Atlas SW, Regenbogen V, Rogers LF, et al: The radiographic characterization of burst fractures of the spine. *AJR* 1986;147;575–582.

3. Bohlman HH: Acute fractures and dislocations of the cervical spine—An analysis of three hundred hospitalized patients and review of the literature. *J Bone Joint Surg* 1979;61A:1119–1142.

4. Braakman R, Penning L: *Injuries of the Cervical Spine*. London, Excerpta Medica, 1971.

5. Cancelmo JJ Jr: Clay shoveler's fracture: A helpful diagnostic sign. *AJR* 1972;115:540–543.

6. Chance GQ: Note on a type of flexion fracture of the spine. *Br J Radiol* 1948;21:452–453.

7. Daffner RH, Deeb ZL, Rothfus WE: ''Fingerprints'' of vertebral trauma—A unifying concept based on mechanisms. *Skeletal Radiol* 1986;15:518–525.

8. Daffner RH, Deeb ZL, Rothfus WE: Thoracic fractures and dislocations in motorcyclists. *Skeletal Radiol* 1987;16:280–284.

9. Dehner JR: Seat belt injuries of the spine and abdomen. *AJR* 1971;111:833–843.

10. Harris JH Jr: Radiographic evaluation of spinal trauma. *Orthop Clin North Am* 1986;17:75–86.

11. Harris JH Jr, Edeiken-Monroe B: *The Radiology of Acute Cervical Spine Trauma*, ed 2. Baltimore, Williams & Wilkins, 1987.

12. Holdsworth FW: Review article: Fractures, dislocations, and fracture-dislocations of the spine. *J Bone Joint Surg* 1970;52A:1534–1551.

13. Roaf R: A study of the mechanics of spinal injuries. *J Bone Joint Surg* 1960;42B:810–823.

14. Smith WS, Kaufer H: Patterns and mechanisms of lumbar injuries associated with lap seatbelts. *J Bone Joint Surg* 1969;51A:239–254.

KEY TO ABBREVIATIONS FOR FIGURES 2-1–2-31

Aa anterior arch of atlas
Ap articular pillar
B body
C central tubercle of atlas
D dens
F foramen transversarium
Ia inferior articular facet
If intervertebral foramen
L lamina
Lm lateral mass
M mammillary process

P pedicle
Pa posterior arch of atlas
Pi pars interarticularis
R rib facet
S spinous process
Sa superior articular facet
Sl spinolaminar line
T transverse process
U uncinate process
V vertebral canal

KEY TO ABBREVIATIONS FOR FIGURES 2-36–2-39

Af articular facet
Al arcuate line
S sacral spine

Sc sacral canal
Sf sacral foramen
Sl sacroiliac joint

Chapter 2

Anatomic Considerations

The vertebral column comprises 33 irregular bones that extend from the base of the skull through the entire length of the neck and trunk. With the attachment of muscles, ligaments, and intervertebral disks, the column forms a strong, flexible support for the body while affording protection for the spinal cord and its surrounding meninges. The column may be divided into the upper 24 presacral vertebrae, which remain separate throughout life, and the fixed vertebrae, which comprise the 5 sacral and 4 coccygeal segments. Although a detailed explanation of the anatomy is beyond the scope of this text, an understanding of the basic anatomic features of the vertebral column is necessary to appreciate the abnormalities that may be encountered in the "spine-injured patient." Those readers who desire a detailed treatment of the anatomy are referred specifically to *The Radiology of Vertebral Trauma*[5] or to a basic textbook on anatomy.[1,6]

BONES

All the movable presacral vertebrae, except for the atlas (C-1) and the axis (C-2), have certain common characteristics. These characteristics constitute the "typical" vertebra. The basic parts of a vertebra are (1) the body, which is weight bearing and located anteriorly; and (2) the vertebral arch, which acts as a protective shell for the spinal cord and its meninges and blood vessels and is located posteriorly. The vertebral arch comprises two pedicles and two laminae. The pedicles attach the arch to the vertebral body. The laminae join the pedicles and form the posterior wall of the vertebral foramen, which encloses the spinal cord and its coverings and vessels. The vertebral arch supports seven projections or processes: two transverse processes, one spinous process, and four articular processes. The transverse processes and spinous process serve as levers on which muscles pull. The articular processes determine the direction and degree of motion of the vertebral column (Fig 2-1).[1,2,4–6,8]

Cervical Vertebrae

The cervical vertebral column may be divided into typical and atypical vertebrae. Vertebrae C-3 through C-6 constitute the typical vertebrae and C-1, C-2, and C-7 the atypical vertebrae. All cervical vertebrae have, as a distinguishing feature, a transverse foramen in each of the transverse processes.[5,6]

In the typical cervical vertebra (Figs 2-2 to 2-7), the vertebral body is elliptical in shape and wider in its transverse diameter than in its sagittal diameter. The upper surface of these vertebrae has a slightly convex appearance from front to back and a concave appearance transversely because of the

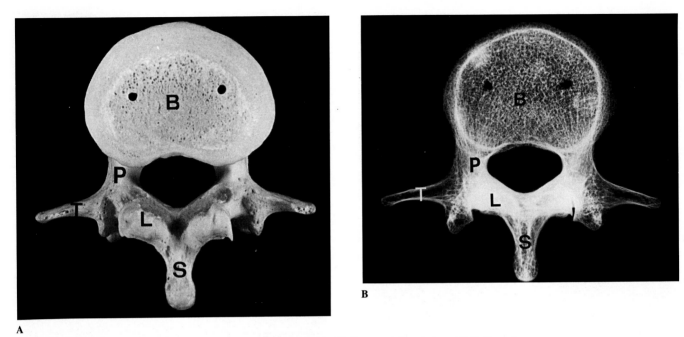

A

B

Figure 2-1 Parts of a ''generic'' vertebra (L-2) (see Key for abbreviations). **(A)** Photograph from below. **(B)** Radiograph.

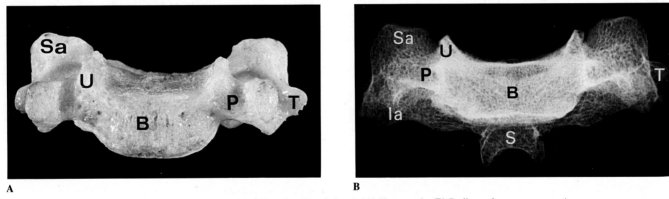

A

B

Figure 2-2 Typical cervical vertebra (C-5), frontal view (see Key for abbreviations). **(A)** Photograph. **(B)** Radiograph.

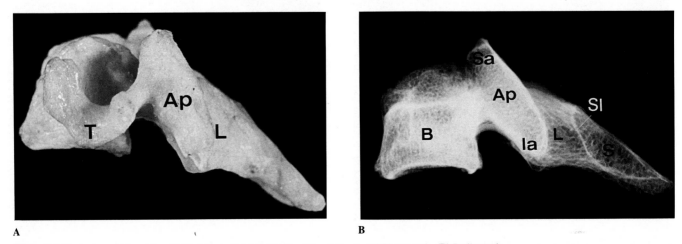

A

B

Figure 2-3 Typical cervical vertebra (C-5), lateral view (see Key for abbreviations). **(A)** Photograph. **(B)** Radiograph.

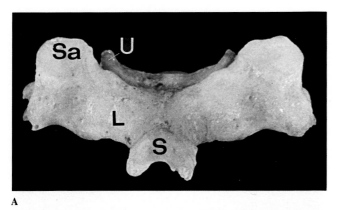
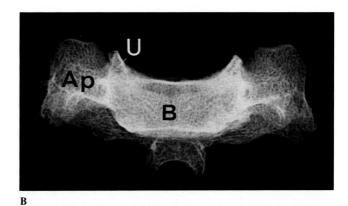

A   **B**

Figure 2-4 Typical cervical vertebra (C-5), posterior view (see Key for abbreviations). **(A)** Photograph. **(B)** Radiograph.

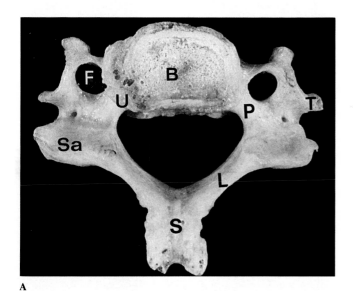
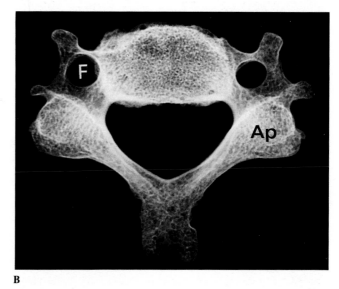

A   **B**

Figure 2-5 Typical cervical vertebra (C-5), view from above (see Key for abbreviations). **(A)** Photograph. **(B)** Radiograph.

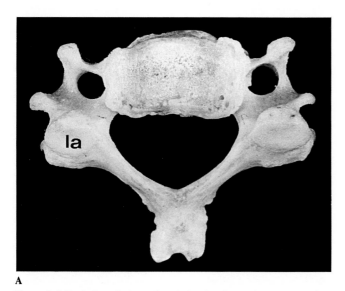
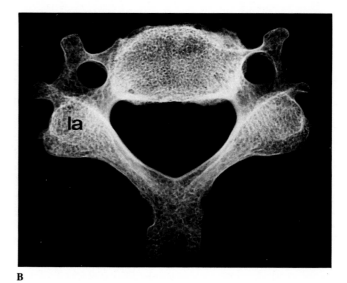

A   **B**

Figure 2-6 Typical cervical vertebra (C-5), view from below (see Key for abbreviations). **(A)** Photograph. **(B)** Radiograph.

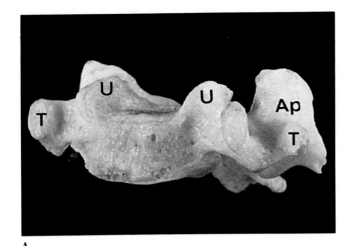

A

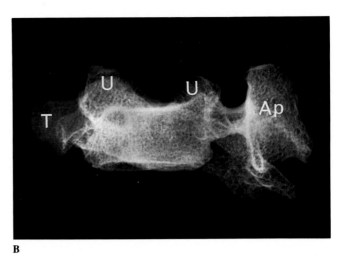

B

Figure 2-7 Typical cervical vertebra (C-5), oblique view (see Key for abbreviations). **(A)** Photograph. **(B)** Radiograph.

presence of the uncinate processes. The superior-anterior surface is beveled to receive the protruding rim of the anterior-inferior surface of the body above. Conversely, the posterior-inferior surface of the body is concave in its sagittal direction and convex transversely to accommodate the uncinate processes of the vertebra below.[1,5,6]

Uncinate processes are not present at birth but develop during adolescence, reaching full height in the adult. Anthropomorphically they are believed to prevent lateral displacement during cervical motion. They project cranially from the upper lateral margins of the posterior aspect of the vertebral bodies of C-3 through C-6 and are found along the posterolateral upper margin of C-7 and T-1.[1,2,4–6]

The cervical pedicles are short and stout and arise from the posterolateral aspect of the vertebral body. They are directed posteriorly and laterally. Typically, they are notched equally on both superior and inferior surfaces.[5]

The laminae are narrow and thin. When viewed on an oblique radiograph, the inferior borders of the laminae overlap the superior aspect of their neighbors like shingles on a roof. This has been termed imbrication.[1,5,6]

The ring formed by the laminae, pedicles, and vertebral body is called the vertebral foramen, which has a triangular shape in the cervical region.[1,5,6]

The superior and inferior articular processes sit on either side of a rhomboid-shaped articular pillar. The pillars project laterally from the junction point of the lamina and pedicle. Each articular process contains a facet that articulates with its neighbor.

The spinous processes are short and directed posteriorly and inferiorly. Typically they are bifid in Caucasians and single in Blacks. Similarly, the transverse processes are short and thin and point inferiorly. This makes it possible to distinguish easily a cervical transverse process from a thoracic transverse process, which points cephalad.[1,5,6]

All cervical vertebrae have a rounded transverse foramen within each transverse process. In the upper six cervical ver-

tebrae, the vertebral artery and vein and a sympathetic nerve plexus are contained within the transverse foramen. The vertebral artery does not pass through the transverse foramen of C-7. The transverse processes have posterior and anterior roots. The posterior root arises from the junction of the lamina and pedicle. Its tip is bulbous and is referred to as the posterior tubercle. The anterior root of the transverse process also ends in a tubercle called the anterior tubercle. This anterior root is also referred to as the costal process.[1,2,4–6,8]

The atlas (C-1), the axis (C-2), and the seventh cervical vertebrae are considered atypical. The atlas differs from all other cervical vertebrae because it lacks both a body and a spinous process. There are essentially five parts of the ring-shaped atlas. The anterior arch consists of the anterior one-fifth. The posterior arch makes up two-fifths, and the remaining two-fifths consist of the lateral masses (Figs 2-8 to 2-13). The anterior and posterior arches contain central tubercles on their outer surfaces, to which the anterior longitudinal ligament, the nuchal ligament, and several muscles attach, respectively. The posterior surface of the anterior arch is slightly concave and contains in its midportion a smooth, rounded depression that articulates with the dens of C-2. The cranial surface of the posterior arch is grooved to accommodate the vertebral artery as it courses through the transverse foramen to enter the skull.[1,5,6,8,9]

The lateral masses of C-1 are fairly large. They represent the ''body'' of this vertebra. The superior articular facets articulate with the occipital condyles. Inferior articular facets articulate with the superior or articular surface of C-2 and permit rotation of the head at the atlanto-axial joint. There is a small tubercle projecting medially from each lateral mass; this is the site for anchoring of the transverse ligament of the atlas. It is this ligament that serves to hold the dens in position against the anterior arch of the atlas.[1,5,6,8,9]

The transverse processes of the atlas are the longest in the cervical region. They serve as anchoring points for muscles that assist in rotation of the head.

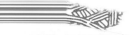

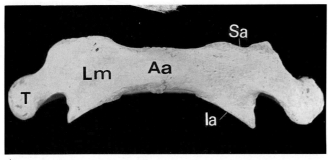

A

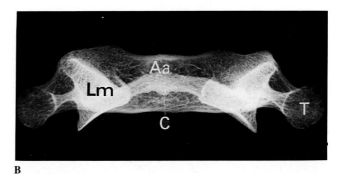

B

Figure 2-8 Atlas (C-1), anterior view (see Key for abbreviations). **(A)** Photograph. **(B)** Radiograph.

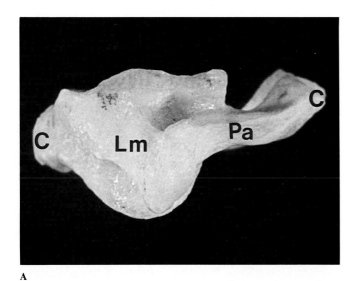

A

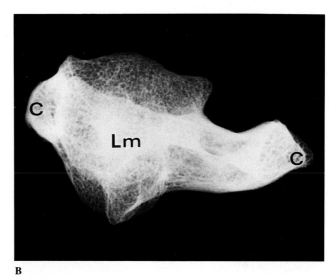

B

Figure 2-9 Atlas (C-1), lateral view (see Key for abbreviations). **(A)** Photograph. **(B)** Radiograph.

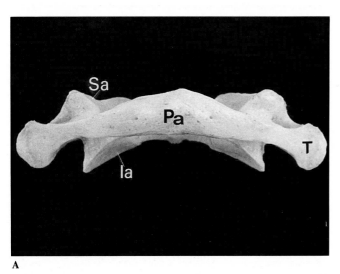

A

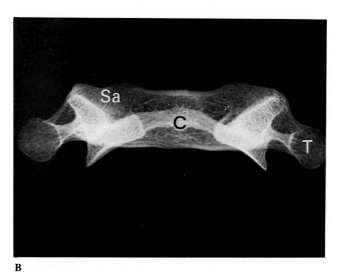

B

Figure 2-10 Atlas (C-1), posterior view (see Key for abbreviations). **(A)** Photograph. **(B)** Radiograph.

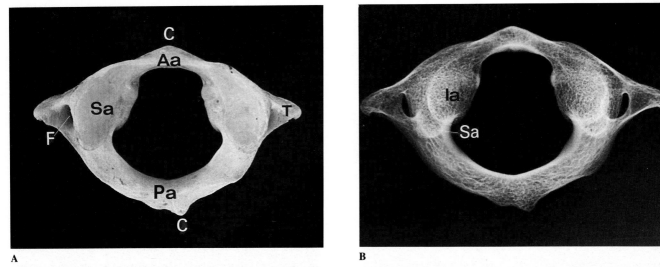

Figure 2-11 Atlas (C-1), view from above (see Key for abbreviations). **(A)** Photograph. **(B)** Radiograph.

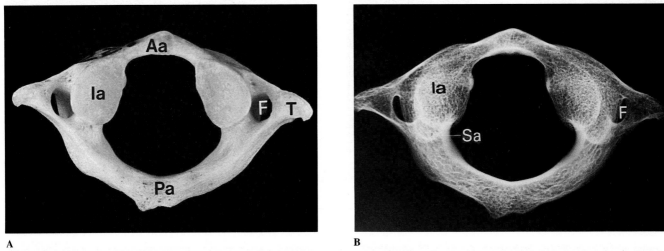

Figure 2-12 Atlas (C-1), view from below (see Key for abbreviations). **(A)** Photograph. **(B)** Radiograph.

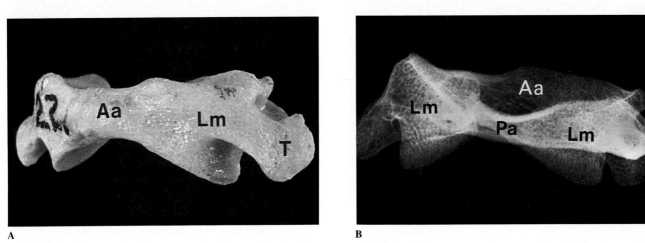

Figure 2-13 Atlas (C-1), oblique view (see Key for abbreviations). **(A)** Photograph. **(B)** Radiograph.

The second cervical vertebra or axis is easily recognized by its toothlike projection (the dens or odontoid process) extending from the upper end of the body (Figs 2-14 to 2-19). There is a distinct narrowing of the dens to form a neck just above the junction of this structure with the body of the axis. The dens contains a rounded facet anteriorly for articulation with the anterior arch of the atlas. Posteriorly, it is grooved to accommodate the transverse ligament of the atlas and a synovial sac.[1,5,6,8,9]

The pedicles of the axis are large and strong. Similarly, the laminae are thick. The superior and inferior articular processes actually extend above and below these areas, and a distinct pars interarticularis may be discerned. The transverse processes are short; the spinous process is also thick.

The seventh cervical vertebra is distinguished by its long, thin, and nonbifid spinous process. This structure may be easily palpated, which explains its other name, the vertebra prominens. The seventh cervical vertebra is further distinguished by a large transverse process that may extend as far laterally as the first thoracic transverse process.[1,5,6,8] Occasionally, a cervical rib may develop from the anterior root of the transverse process (Fig 2-20).

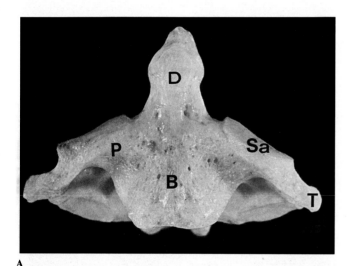

A

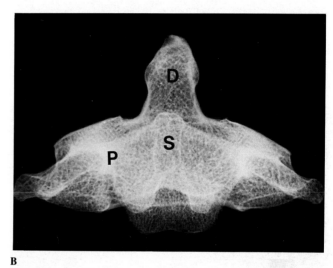

B

Figure 2-14 Axis (C-2), frontal view (see Key for abbreviations). **(A)** Photograph. **(B)** Radiograph.

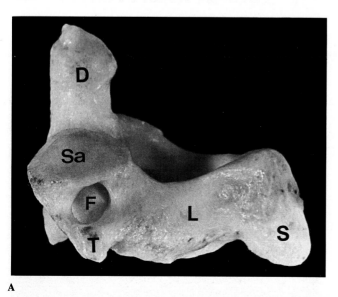

A

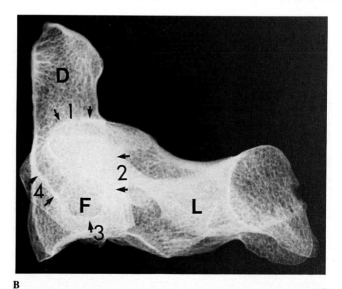

B

Figure 2-15 Axis (C-2), lateral view (see Key for abbreviations). **(A)** Photograph. **(B)** Radiograph. Harris' "ring" is outlined by arrows. This is a composite shadow that is made up of the following structures: (1) the upper margin of the superior articular facet, (2) the posterior aspect of the body of C-2, (3) the inferior border of the transverse foramen, and (4) the pedicle and anterior portion of the body of C-2.

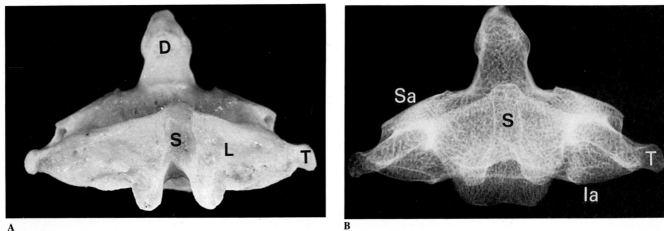

A
B

Figure 2-16 Axis (C-2), posterior view (see Key for abbreviations). **(A)** Photograph. **(B)** Radiograph.

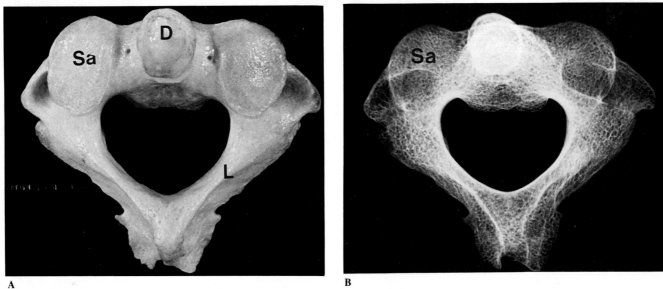

A
B

Figure 2-17 Axis (C-2), view from above (see Key for abbreviations). **(A)** Photograph. **(B)** Radiograph.

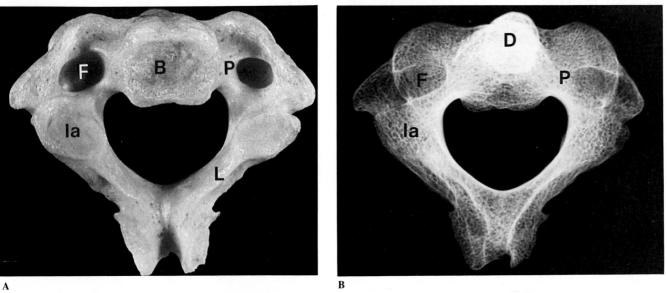

A
B

Figure 2-18 Axis (C-2), view from below (see Key for abbreviations). **(A)** Photograph. **(B)** Radiograph.

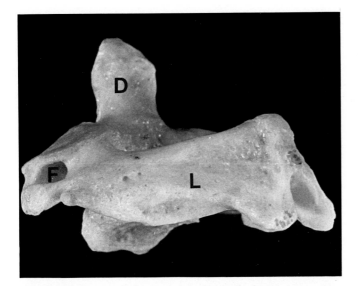

A

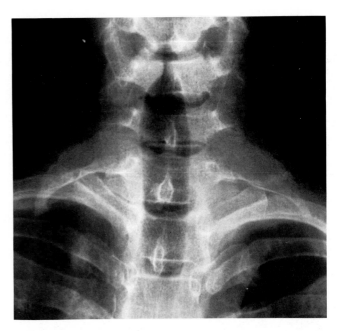

Figure 2-20 Cervical ribs. These anomalous ribs arise from transverse processes that are pointed downward, which identifies their cervical origin. The transverse processes of the thoracic vertebrae all point cephalad.

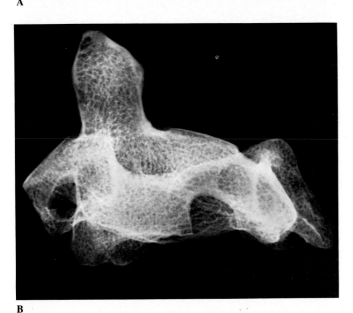

B

Figure 2-19 Axis (C-2), oblique view (see Key for abbreviations). **(A)** Photograph. **(B)** Radiograph.

Thoracic Vertebrae

The 12 thoracic vertebrae are recognized by the presence of costal facets superiorly and inferiorly on each side of the body and along the transverse processes. These facets articulate with the heads and articular tubercles of the ribs. The last two thoracic vertebrae lack facets on their transverse processes. As in the cervical region, there are typical and atypical vertebrae. The second through eighth thoracic vertebrae are considered typical; T-1 and T-9 through T-12 are atypical.[1,5,6]

The typical thoracic vertebra has a reniform shape with a small dorsal waist. Although the transverse and sagittal diameters are approximately equal, they are slightly taller posteri-

orly than anteriorly; this results in the normal thoracic kyphosis. This becomes important when radiographs are analyzed for minimal compression fractures, since the typical vertical height is up to 2 mm less anteriorly than the vertical height posteriorly at the same level.[5] The lateral aspects of the vertebral bodies contain demifacets for articulation with the rib on either side of the disk space. The transverse process, which is long and club-shaped, also contains a facet for articulation with the rib. Similarly, all the typical ribs contain demifacets superiorly and inferiorly and a third facet along their tubercles for articulation with the transverse processes. The articular facet of the neck of any typical rib always articulates with the transverse process of its own numbered vertebra.[1,5,6] This becomes important in evaluating patients who may have suffered shearing or lateral flexion injuries.

The spinous processes of the typical thoracic vertebrae are long and slender and slope inferiorly, overlapping the spine of the vertebra below. There is variation in the degree of slope of the spinous processes; T-1 and T-2 are almost horizontal, T-5 through T-8 are nearly vertical, and T-11 and T-12 are horizontal. Figures 2-21 through 2-25 show a typical thoracic vertebra.

The first thoracic vertebra and the ninth through twelfth thoracic vertebrae are considered atypical.[5] The first thoracic vertebra resembles a cervical vertebra. It is the only thoracic vertebra that contains an uncinate process.[1,5,6] The entire head of the first rib articulates in a full facet along the lateral superior aspect of this vertebra. The ninth and tenth vertebrae

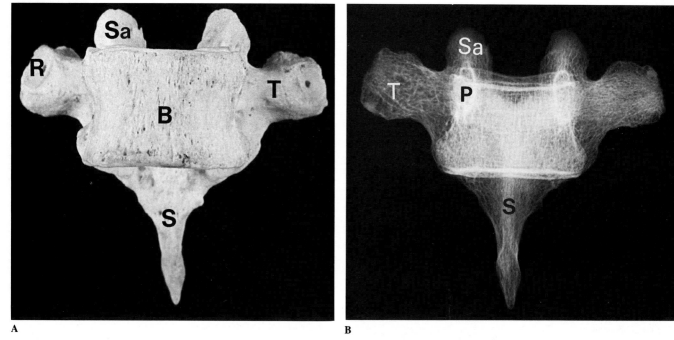

A
B

Figure 2-21 Typical thoracic vertebra (T-7), frontal view (see Key for abbreviations). (**A**) Photograph. (**B**) Radiograph.

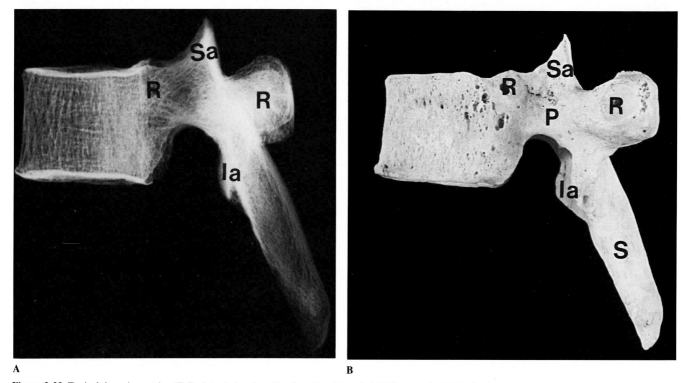

A
B

Figure 2-22 Typical thoracic vertebra (T-7), lateral view (see Key for abbreviations). (**A**) Photograph. (**B**) Radiograph.

vary in the arrangement of their costal facets. Vertebra T-9 has a demifacet superiorly and no facet inferiorly. Vertebra T-10 has a full facet superiorly and no facet inferiorly. Vertebrae T-11 and T-12 resemble lumbar vertebrae; their short trans- verse processes lack facets for rib articulations, and their bodies are quite large.[1,2,4-6] Indeed, absence of ribs from T-12, a common anomaly, may result in mistaken identification of this vertebra as L-1.

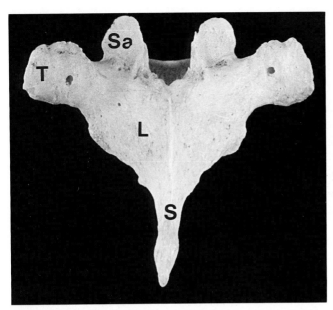

Figure 2-23 Typical thoracic vertebra (T-7), posterior view, photograph (see Key for abbreviations).

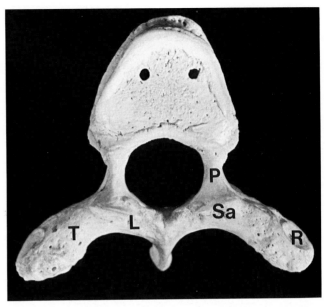

Figure 2-24 Typical thoracic vertebra (T-7), view from above (see Key for abbreviations). (**A**) Photograph.

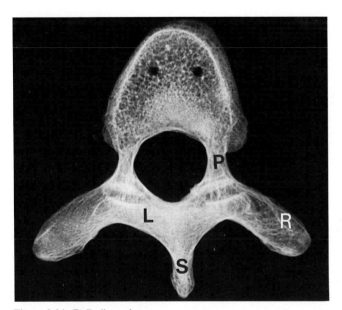

Figure 2-24 (**B**) Radiograph.

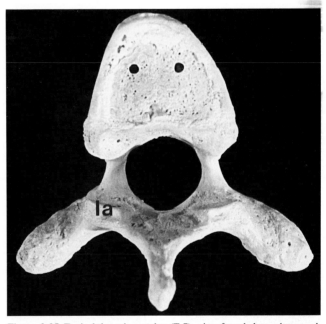

Figure 2-25 Typical thoracic vertebra (T-7), view from below, photograph (see Key for abbreviations).

Lumbar Vertebrae

The lumbar vertebrae are the largest and heaviest segments of the presacral part of the vertebral column (Figs 2-26 to 2-31). These vertebrae are easily distinguished from their mates elsewhere in the column by their lack of costal facets and transverse foramina in their transverse processes. Their spinous processes are large and rectangular; their transverse processes are thin. The typical lumbar vertebral body is large and reniform with a shallow dorsal concavity abutting a triangular vertebral foramen. Like the thoracic vertebrae, the first two lumbar vertebral bodies are taller posteriorly than anteriorly. The reverse is true of the fourth and fifth vertebrae; this results in a lumbar lordosis.[1,2,4–6]

The lumbar pedicles are short and arise from the upper lateral margin of the vertebral bodies. The inferior vertebral

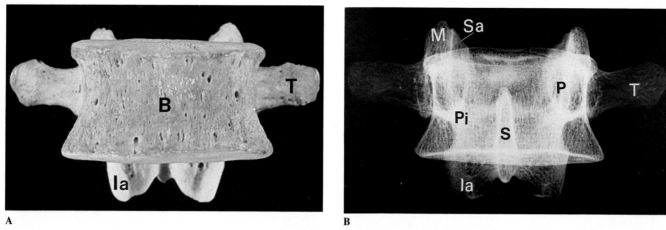

A   **B**

Figure 2-26 Typical lumbar vertebra (L-3), frontal view (see Key for abbreviations). (**A**) Photograph. (**B**) Radiograph.

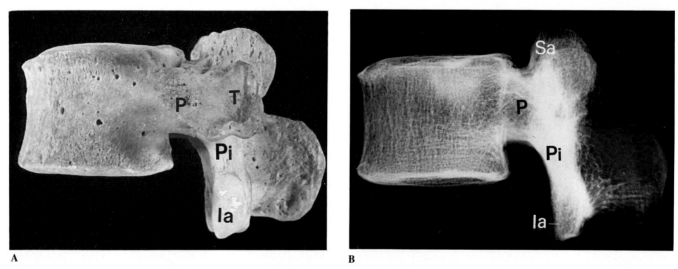

A   **B**

Figure 2-27 Typical lumbar vertebra (L-3), lateral view (see Key for abbreviations). (**A**) Photograph. (**B**) Radiograph.

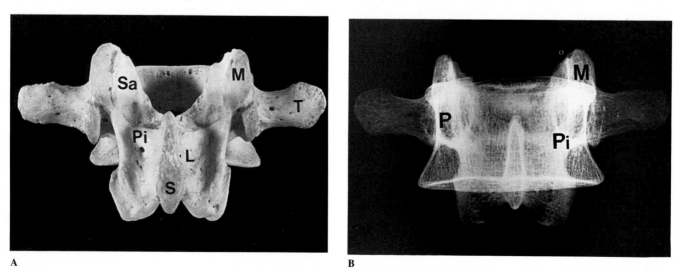

A   **B**

Figure 2-28 Typical lumbar vertebra (L-3), posterior view (see Key for abbreviations). (**A**) Photograph. (**B**) Radiograph.

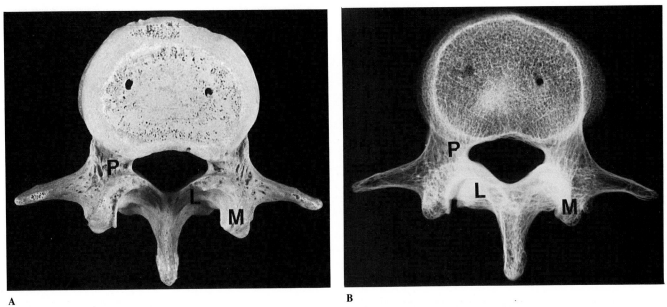

Figure 2-29 Typical lumbar vertebra (L-3), view from above (see Key for abbreviations). (**A**) Photograph. (**B**) Radiograph.

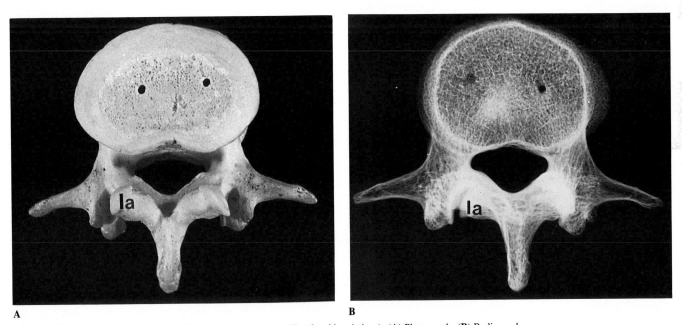

Figure 2-30 Typical lumbar vertebra (L-3), view from below (see Key for abbreviations). (**A**) Photograph. (**B**) Radiograph.

notches are deeper than the superior ones. Similarly, the laminae of the lumbar vertebrae are large and thick. The superior and inferior articular processes project above and below the laminae, respectively, just behind the pedicles. The portion of the lamina between these two processes is known as the pars interarticularis.[1,5,6] It is through this site that spondylolysis occurs (Fig 2-32). There is a small, knobby pro-

tuberance, the mammillary process, extending from the posterolateral tip of each superior articular facet. This structure is for attachment of postvertebral muscles.

The transverse processes are elongated, thin, and flattened. At the base of the transverse process there is a small, rough tubercle known as the accessory process, which is the site of muscle attachment. If the accessory process is greater

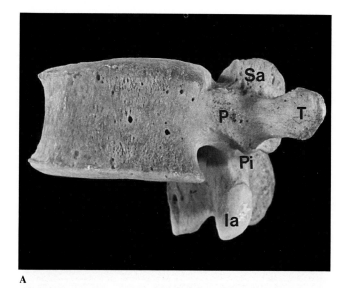

A

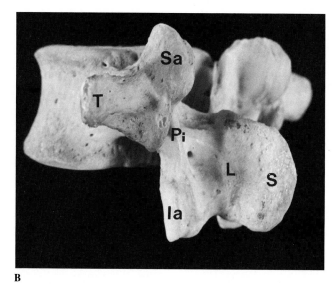

B

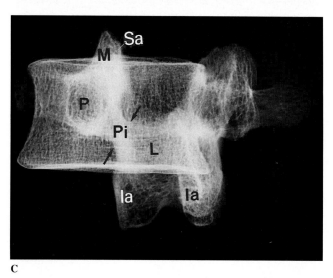

C

Figure 2-31 Typical lumbar vertebra (L-3), oblique view (see Key for abbreviations). (**A**) Anterior oblique photograph of specimen. (**B**) Posterior oblique photograph of specimen. (**C**) Radiograph. Note the appearance of the "Scotty dog." The snout is the transverse process, the eye is the pedicle, the ear is the superior articular facet and the mammillary process, the neck is the pars interarticularis (arrows), the body is the lamina, and the feet are the inferior articular processes.

than 5 mm in length, it is termed the styloid process (Fig 2-33).[1,2,4-6]

There are a number of anomalies that occur in the thoracolumbar and lumbosacral areas that occasionally result in confusion regarding the numbering of lumbar vertebrae. These common anomalies include absence of the twelfth rib, presence of a first lumbar rib, sacralization of L-5 (Fig 2-34), and lumbarization of the first sacral segment (Fig 2-35).[4,5,8] These anomalies present diagnostic difficulties when it is absolutely necessary to be able to identify a particular vertebral level for site of injury, site of myelographic abnormality, or site of surgical intervention.

When such an anomaly is encountered, there are three methods that may be used to determine the correct lumbar levels. The first method requires the availability of a chest radiograph or thoracic vertebral radiograph. If such a study is available, it is a simple task to count the thoracic vertebrae. If there are no other films available, the second method should be used. This method is based on the fact that a line drawn across the iliac crests passes through or near the L-4 intervertebral disk space. The third method relies on the fact that the transverse processes of L-3 are the most horizontal and are usually the longest.[5]

Occasionally, it is impossible to identify a lumbar level with confidence by any method. In these unusual circumstances, it is best to identify the level of abnormality by counting from the last rib-bearing vertebra. For example, if the radiologist tells the surgeon that there is a burst fracture involving the second non-rib-bearing vertebra, the clinician has a definite point of reference.

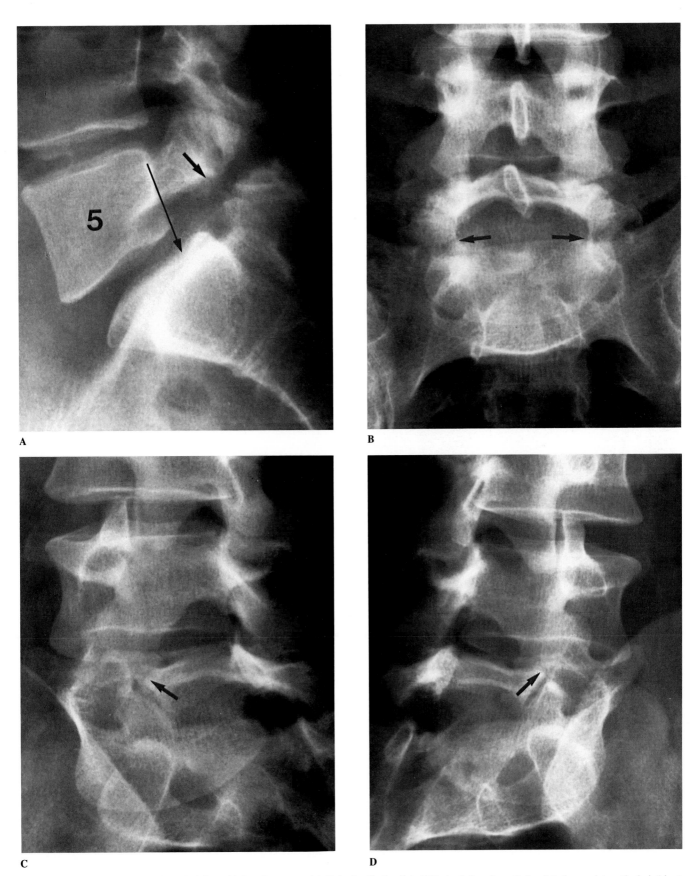

Figure 2-32 Bilateral pars interarticularis defect with first-degree spondylolisthesis of L-5 on S-1. (**A**) Lateral view shows the break in the pars interarticularis (short arrow). Note the anterolisthesis of L-5 on S-1 (long arrow). (**B**) Frontal view shows the bilateral pars defects (arrows) in L-5. (**C and D**) Oblique radiographs do not show the pars defects at L-5 (arrows) as well as the lateral film. Compare with the vertebrae above L-5.

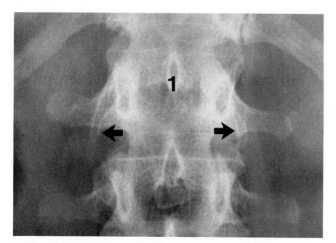

Figure 2-33 Lumbar styloid processes of L-1 (arrows).

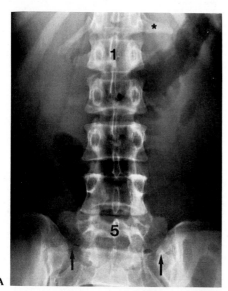

A

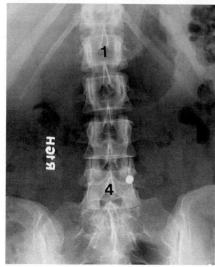

B

Figure 2-34 Sacralization of L-5. A line drawn across the iliac crests should pass through the L4-5 junction. (A) There are broad transverse processes of L-5 with assimilation joints between L-5 and S-1 (arrows). There is an anomalous rib of T-12 on the left (*). (B) Another patient with complete sacralization of L-5.

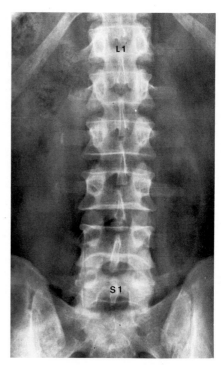

Figure 2-35 Lumbarization of the first sacral segment. This patient has six non-rib-bearing vertebrae. Her chest radiograph showed 12 rib-bearing thoracic vertebrae.

Sacrum and Coccyx

The sacrum comprises five sacral vertebrae fused in the adult to form a wedge-shaped bone (Figs 2-36 to 2-39). The sacrum articulates with the iliac bones laterally, and its base articulates with the last lumbar vertebra. The coccyx attaches inferiorly. The pelvic surface of the sacrum is concave. Along the pelvic surface are four transverse ridges that form the pelvic sacral foramina. The superior aspect of these foramina is easily recognizable on frontal radiographs as a thin, archlike density. These are referred to as the sacral arcuate lines (Fig 2-36). These lines are important in diagnosing occult sacral fractures (Fig 2-40).[1,2,4–6,8]

The coccyx is formed by four rudimentary vertebrae. Injuries to the coccyx generally present no difficulties from the standpoint of radiologic diagnosis.

JOINTS AND LIGAMENTS

The vertebral column is articulated through a series of joints and supporting ligaments. There are two series of joints that unite the individual vertebrae; the only exceptions are the joints between the occiput and the atlas and between the atlas and the axis, owing to their special anatomy.[9] There are essentially two types of joints: slightly movable (amphi-

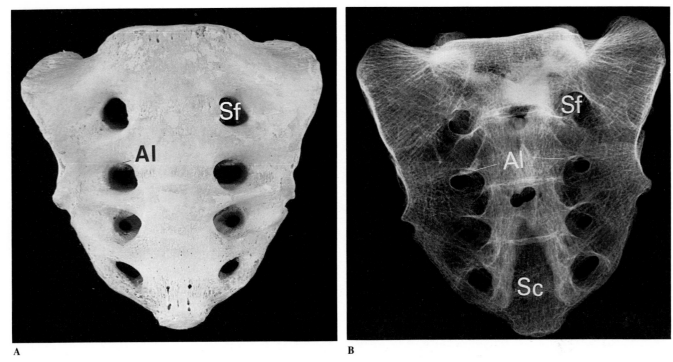

Figure 2-36 Sacrum, frontal view (see Key to abbreviations). (**A**) Photograph. (**B**) Radiograph.

KEY TO ABBREVIATIONS FOR FIGURES 2-36–2-39

Af	articular facet	**Sc**	sacral canal
Al	arcuate line	**Sf**	sacral foramen
S	sacral spine	**Sl**	sacroiliac joint

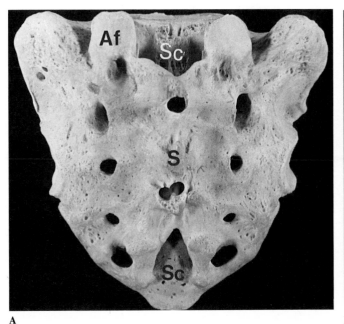
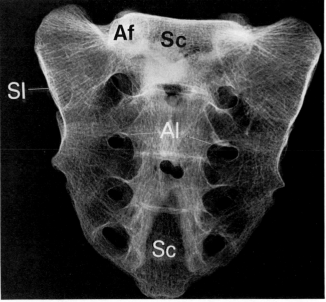

Figure 2-37 Sacrum, posterior view (see Key to abbreviations). (**A**) Photograph. (**B**) Radiograph.

arthrodial) symphyseal joints, and freely movable (diarthrodial) synovial joints (Fig 2-41). The intervertebral disks are typical amphiarthrodial joints. The apophyseal joints or facet joints are diarthrodial joints that are enclosed in a fibrous capsule lined by synovial membrane. Motion in these joints is of a gliding nature, and the surfaces of the joints are relatively flat.[7] Hence movement is permitted by laxity in the articular capsule and is limited by the ligaments and osseous structures surrounding the joint. Motion about the disk spaces is markedly limited and is dependent mainly on disk thickness. Thus

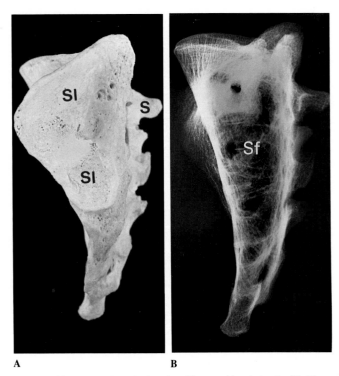

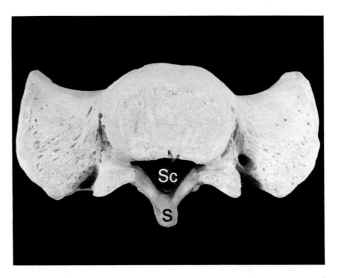

Figure 2-39 Sacrum, view from above, photograph (see Key to abbreviations).

A   **B**

Figure 2-38 Sacrum, lateral view (see Key to abbreviations). (**A**) Photograph. (**B**) Radiograph.

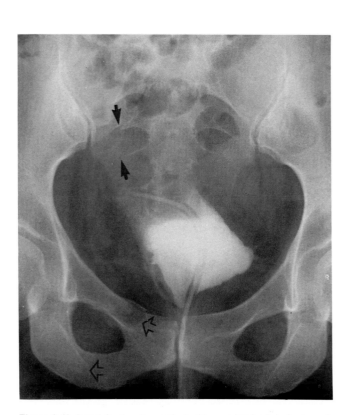

Figure 2-40 Sacral fracture in a patient with associated pelvic fracture. A frontal view of the pelvis shows interruption of the sacral arcuate lines on the right (short arrows). In addition, there are fractures of the ischiopubic arches on the right side (open arrows). Note the pelvic hematoma displacing the contrast-filled bladder to the left. There is gas in the extraperitoneal soft tissues as a result of extraperitoneal bladder rupture.

the greatest degree of motion is present in the cervical and lumbar regions, where the disks are the thickest.

Intervertebral disks comprise anatomically a laminated outer portion, the anulus fibrosis, and an inner portion, the nucleus pulposus (Fig 2-42).[1,2,4–6,8] Both these structures derive embryologically from notochordal remnants. The nucleus pulposus is eccentrically located when viewed in the sagittal plane, and the shorter distance to the vertebral canal accounts for the more common herniation of this material into the canal than anteriorly.

In the cervical region, synovial joints between the uncinate processes and the intervertebral disks are present and are referred to as Luschka's or uncovertebral joints. There is some controversy regarding whether or not they are true joints. Most authorities now believe that they are actually fissures without true synovial linings.[4,5,8] Because the uncinate processes are not present at birth, these joints develop as the individual grows. As in true synovial joints, however, osteophytes develop in response to stress in these regions and may encroach on nerves leaving the intervertebral foramina.

The vertebral bodies are linked by two strong ligamentous bands (Fig 2-43). The anterior longitudinal ligament is located over the anterolateral surfaces of the vertebral bodies. It is thinnest at its attachment to the base of skull at the occipital bone. It is also thicker in the thoracic region than in the cervical or lumbar regions and is thickest over the central concavity of each vertebral body, where it actually blends with the periosteum.[5,6]

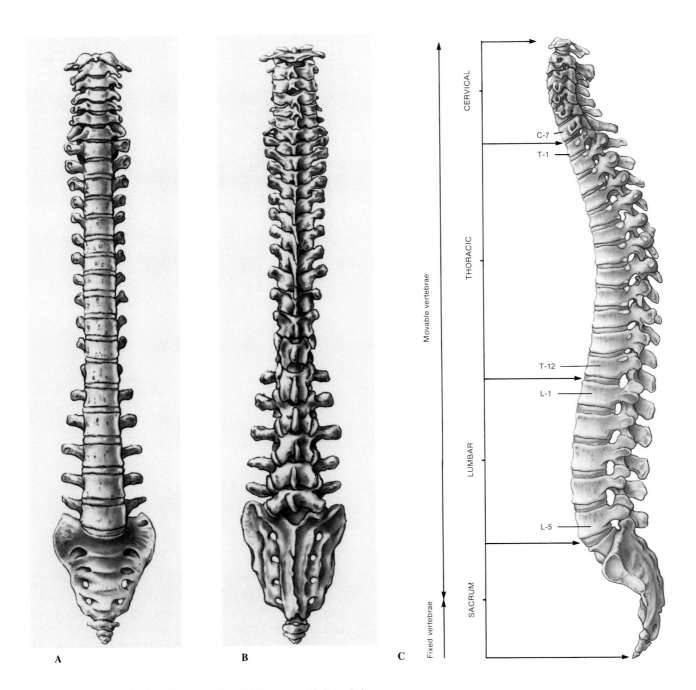

Figure 2-41 Articulated spine. (**A**) Frontal view. (**B**) Rear view. (**C**) Lateral view.

The posterior longitudinal ligament is on the posterior surface of the vertebral bodies within the vertebral canal (Fig 2-43). In the cervical region it attaches to the body of the axis and becomes continuous with the tectorial membrane. The posterior longitudinal ligament is firmly bound to the intervertebral disks. This is in contradistinction to the anterior longitudinal ligament, which is not intimately bound to the same extent. It is separated from the vertebral bodies by the venous plexuses, however.[5,6]

Posterior to the vertebral bodies are the apophyseal joints, which are the important articulation (Fig 2-43).[5,6,8] These are true synovial joints that are surrounded by a thin fibrous capsule attached to the outer surfaces of the articular processes. Unlike the fibrocartilage of the intervertebral disk space, the articular processes are covered by thin hyaline cartilage.

Posterior support to the vertebral column is given by the ligamenta flava and by the supraspinal ligament (Fig 2-43).

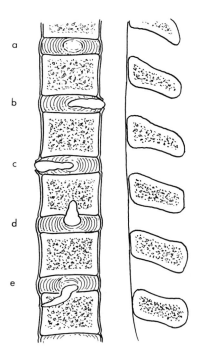

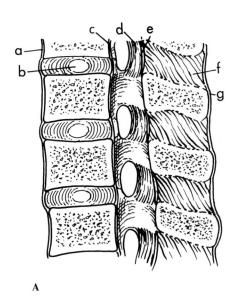

A

Figure 2-42 Schematic drawing of the intervertebral disk space. The intervertebral disk comprises the anulus fibrosis and the nucleus pulposus (a). Disruption of the diskovertebral joint may result in posterior herniation of nuclear material (b), anterior herniation (c), intraosseous herniation to produce a Schmorl's nodule (d), or anteroinferior herniation to produce a vertebral edge separation (e). *Source:* Reprinted from ''Injuries of the Thoracolumbar Vertebral Column'' by RH Daffner in *Radiology in Emergency Medicine* by MK Dalinka and JJ Kaye (Eds) with permission of Churchill Livingstone Inc, © 1984.

Figure 2-43 Vertebral ligaments. (**A**) Schematic overview in sagittal section [(a) anterior longitudinal ligament, (b) nucleus pulposus, (c) posterior longitudinal ligament, (d) interfacet joint ligament, (e) ligamentum flavum, (f) interspinous ligament, (g) supraspinous ligament.] *Source:* Reprinted from ''Injuries of the Thoracolumbar Vertebral Column'' by RH Daffner in *Radiology in Emergency Medicine* by MK Dalinka and JJ Kaye (Eds) with permission of Churchill Livingstone Inc, © 1984.

The ligamenta flava are actually paired ligaments connecting the laminae. They arise from the anterior surface of the lower lamina and attach to the upper portion of the posterior surface of the next succeeding lamina. They are separated in the midline by venous structures.

The supraspinal ligament is composed of thin layers of fibrous tissue coursing over the tips of the spinous processes. There is variation in the attachment of these ligamentous fibers. Shorter fibers connect adjacent spinous processes, and longer ones connect several vertebrae. In the lumbar region, deep fibers merge with those of the interspinal ligament laterally. In the cervical region, the supraspinal ligament becomes part of the nuchal ligament.[9] Ossification may occur within the nuchal ligament (Fig 2-44).

The interspinal ligament is a thin structure extending between adjacent spinous processes. Degeneration may occur with aging, and osteoarthrosis (Baastrup's disease) may occur, particularly in the lumbar region (Fig 2-45).

The inherent stability of the vertebral column depends on the integrity of these ligamentous structures and adjacent bones. Denis proposed a three-column approach to determin-

ing vertebral stability.[3] The anterior column lies between the anterior longitudinal ligament and a vertical line through the midportion of the vertebral body. The middle column extends from this line to the posterior longitudinal ligament. The posterior column extends through the posterior arch of the vertebra to the supraspinal ligament (Fig 2-43). According to Denis, disruption of any single column will not result in instability.[3] Disruption of two contiguous columns, however, produces instability. This will be discussed in greater depth in Chapter 4.

The atlanto-axial articulation is complex and consists of three joints: a middle atlanto-axial joint and two paired lateral joints (Figs 2-46 to 2-48). The middle atlanto-axial joint is a pivot type of joint with two small synovial sacs on either side of the dens; the posterior synovial sac is the larger of the two. Except for their size, the lateral atlanto-axial joints are quite similar to facet joints found elsewhere in the vertebral column.[9]

The tectorial membrane is a broad band of fiber that extends from the posterior longitudinal ligament along the lower aspect of the body of C-2 and stretches cranially to attach to the inner aspect of the base of the occiput (Figs 2-49 and 2-50). It

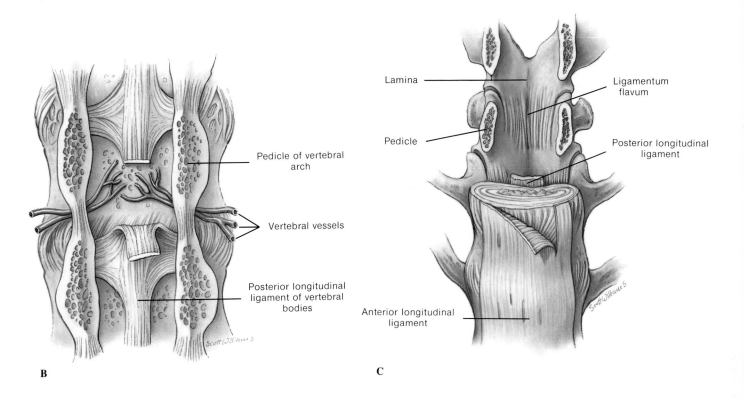

B

Pedicle of vertebral arch

Vertebral vessels

Posterior longitudinal ligament of vertebral bodies

C

Lamina

Pedicle

Anterior longitudinal ligament

Ligamentum flavum

Posterior longitudinal ligament

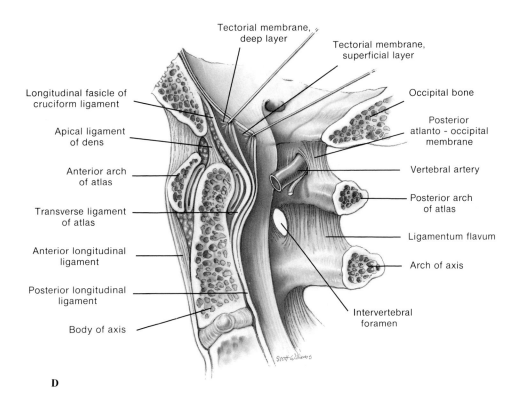

Tectorial membrane, deep layer

Tectorial membrane, superficial layer

Longitudinal fasicle of cruciform ligament

Apical ligament of dens

Anterior arch of atlas

Transverse ligament of atlas

Anterior longitudinal ligament

Posterior longitudinal ligament

Body of axis

Occipital bone

Posterior atlanto - occipital membrane

Vertebral artery

Posterior arch of atlas

Ligamentum flavum

Arch of axis

Intervertebral foramen

D

Figure 2-43 (**B**) The posterior longitudinal ligament, view from behind. The vertebra has been sectioned at the level of the pedicles. The posterior longitudinal ligament has been retracted to reveal the vertebral veins. (**C**) Vertebral ligaments, view from the front. The vertebra has been sectioned through an intervertebral disk and through the pedicles. The anterior longitudinal ligament is retracted. The ligamentum flavum is clearly visible. (**D**) Sagittal section shows relation of the various ligaments at the craniovertebral junction.

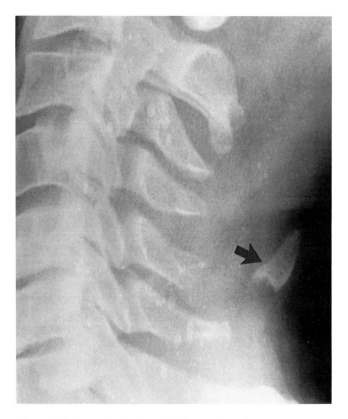

covers the dens and the other ligaments. Just anterior to the tectorial membrane is the cruciform ligament. It has two components, a transverse portion (the transverse ligament) and a vertical portion. The transverse ligament attaches to the small turbercles on the medial sides of the lateral masses of C-1. This ligament holds the dens against the anterior arch of the atlas. A synovial sac is located between the transverse ligament and the dens.[5,9]

The atlanto-occipital joint is also complex and is formed by the convex occipital condyle and the concave superior articular surface of the atlas (Figs 2-49 and 2-50). These joints are enclosed by a synovial-lined articular capsule. The fibrous anterior atlanto-occipital membrane and posterior atlanto-occipital membrane are quite broad, and the anterior membrane is the denser of the two. The posterior membrane is analogous to the ligamentum flavum in its relationship to the vertebral canal. It adheres to the posterior margin of the foramen magnum and also to the posterior arch of the atlas.[5,9]

The sacroiliac joints comprise a true synovial joint anteriorly and a fibrous joint posteriorly. Accessory ligaments bolster the strength of the sacroiliac joint and provide sacroiliac stability (Figs 2-51 and 2-52).

Figure 2-44 Ossification in the nuchal ligament (arrow).

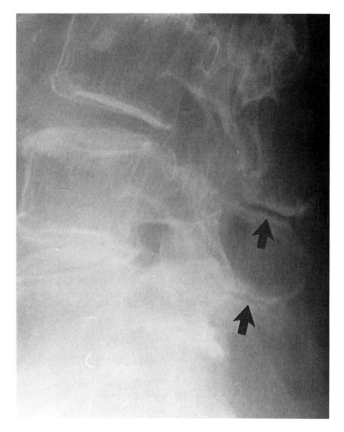

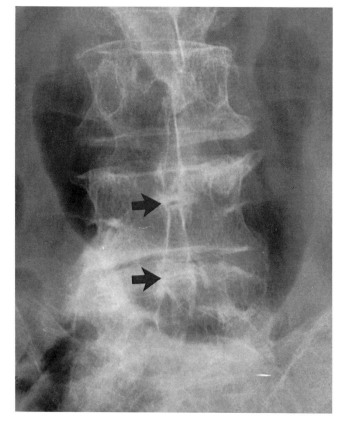

Figure 2-45 Degenerative change between spinous processes (Baastrup's disease) (arrows).

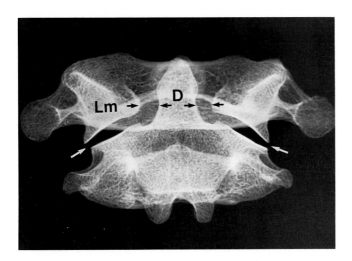

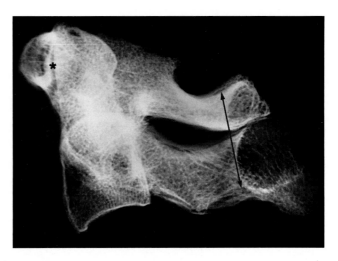

Figure 2-46 The atlanto-axial articulation, frontal view. In particular, note the relationship of the lateral masses of C-1 (Lm) and their articulation to the body of C-2. Under normal circumstances, there should never be more than 2 mm of unilateral or bilateral atlanto-axial overlap at the point indicated by white arrows. Similarly, there should be never more than 2 mm between the lateral margins of the dens (D) and the medial margins of the lateral masses of C-1 (small arrows).

Figure 2-47 Atlanto-axial joint, lateral view. Prevertebral space (*) should never exceed 3 mm in an adult and 5 mm in a child. The spinolaminar line (long arrow) should be smooth and uninterrupted.

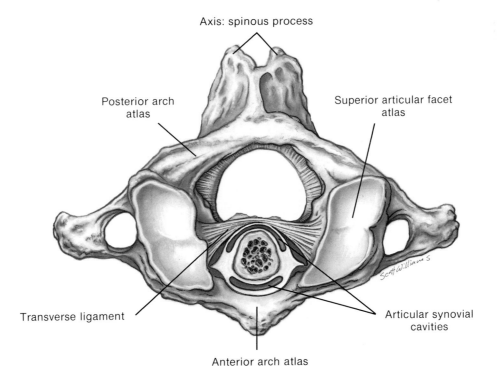

Figure 2-48 The altanto-axial joint, view from above.

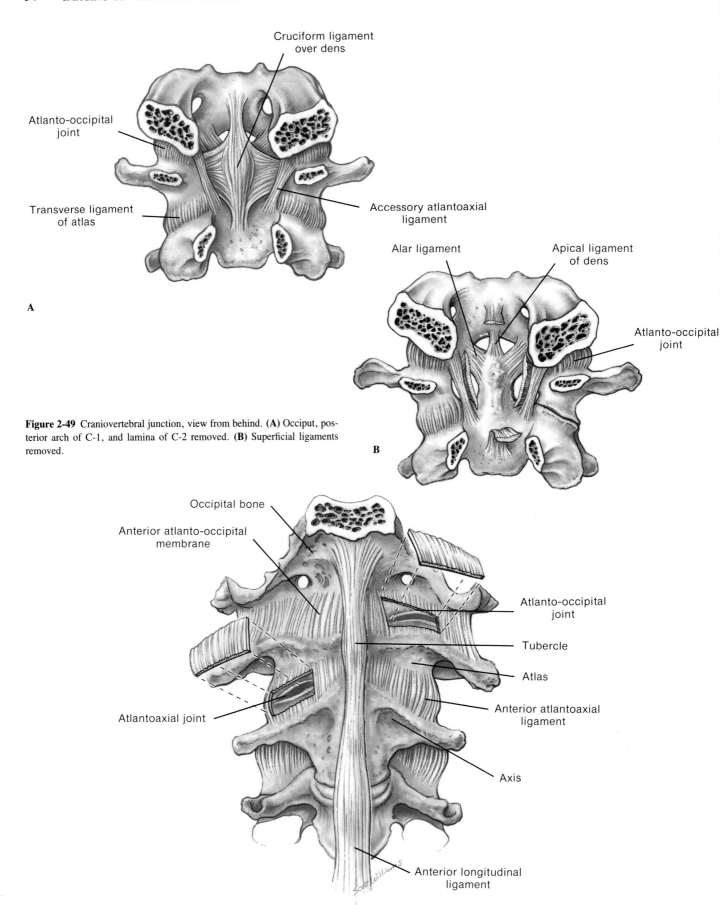

Figure 2-49 Craniovertebral junction, view from behind. **(A)** Occiput, posterior arch of C-1, and lamina of C-2 removed. **(B)** Superficial ligaments removed.

Figure 2-50 Craniovertebral junction, view fruom the front (for a sagittal view see Fig 2-43D).

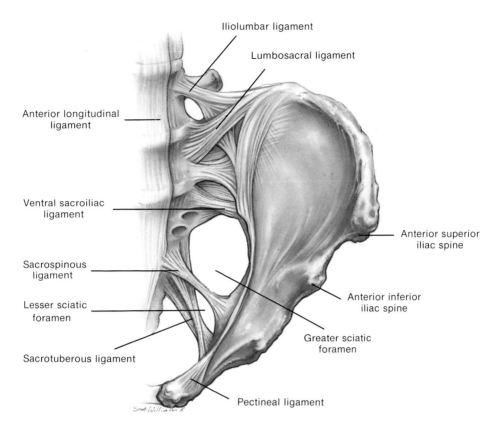

Iliolumbar ligament

Lumbosacral ligament

Anterior longitudinal ligament

Ventral sacroiliac ligament

Sacrospinous ligament

Lesser sciatic foramen

Sacrotuberous ligament

Anterior superior iliac spine

Anterior inferior iliac spine

Greater sciatic foramen

Pectineal ligament

Figure 2-51 The sacroiliac joint, view from the front.

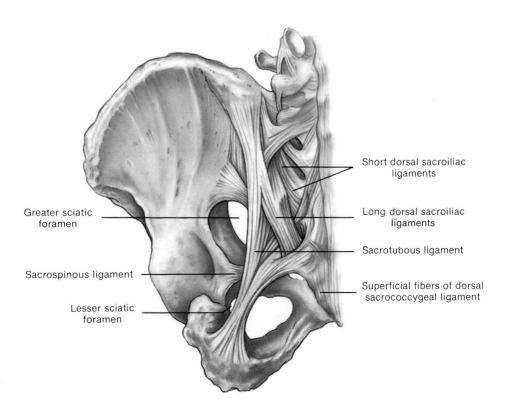

Short dorsal sacroiliac ligaments

Long dorsal sacroiliac ligaments

Sacrotubous ligament

Superficial fibers of dorsal sacrococcygeal ligament

Greater sciatic foramen

Sacrospinous ligament

Lesser sciatic foramen

Figure 2-52 The sacroiliac joint, view from behind.

REFERENCES

1. Anderson JE: *Grant's Atlas of Anatomy*, ed 8. Baltimore, Williams & Wilkins, 1983, pp 5-1–5-23.

2. Banna M: *Clinical Radiology of the Spine and the Spinal Cord.* Rockville, Md, Aspen Publishers Inc, 1985, pp 1–158.

3. Denis F: The three column spine and its significance in the classification of acute thoracolumbar spinal injuries. *Spine* 1983;8:817–831.

4. Epstein BS: *The Spine: A Radiologic Text and Atlas,* ed 4. Philadelphia, Lea & Febiger, 1976.

5. Gehweiler JA Jr, Osborne RL Jr, Becker RF: *The Radiology of Vertebral Trauma.* Philadelphia, WB Saunders, 1980, pp 3–88.

6. Goss, CM: *Gray's Anatomy of the Human Body*, ed 29 (American). Philadelphia, Lea & Febiger, 1973, pp 100–121, 294–305.

7. Penning L: Normal movements of the cervical spine. *AJR* 1978;130:317–326.

8. Schmorl G, Junghanns H: *The Human Spine in Health and Disease,* ed 5. New York, Grune & Stratton, 1971.

9. Von Torklus D, Gehle W: *The Upper Cervical Spine: Regional Anatomy, Pathology, and Traumatology: A Systematic Radiological Atlas and Textbook.* New York, Grune & Stratton, 1972.

Chapter 3

Imaging for Vertebral Trauma

The referring physician and radiologist have many imaging techniques available to diagnose the extent of vertebral injury. These include plain film radiography, computed tomography (CT), conventional polydirectional tomography (PT), magnetic resonance (MR), and myelography. These techniques are used alone or in combinations to arrive at the correct diagnosis. This chapter reviews each of these imaging formats and illustrates its use in the diagnosis of vertebral injury. Chapters 4 and 5 describe the integrated use of multiple imaging techniques.

PLAIN FILM RADIOGRAPHY

Plain film radiography is the foundation on which the diagnosis of vertebral injuries should be made.[10,15,16] In an era when specialized imaging techniques such as CT and MR are quite commonplace studies, plain film radiography has been given less emphasis. Nevertheless, a proper diagnosis cannot be made in most instances unless basic diagnostic information is obtained. This author makes extensive use of plain film radiography and relies on it to make an initial diagnosis. Special imaging techniques are then used to confirm the initial impression and to outline the extent of damage. Furthermore, the author considers it bad medical and radiologic practice to perform a specialized imaging study without the use of plain films for guidance.

Techniques

What is the "routine" series of radiographs for examining a patient with an acute vertebral injury? This question is frequently asked of radiologists by their surgical colleagues. Although there are differing opinions as to which views should be routine, a practical approach may be adopted. In our institution we utilize the series shown in Table 3-1.

Table 3-1 "Routine" Examination for Suspected Vertebral Injury

1. Cervical column
   - lateral-horizontal beam
   - anterior-posterior (AP) of the lower cervical column
   - AP of the atlas-axis
   - trauma oblique views
   - upright lateral before discharge
   - lateral flexion-extension views if needed
2. Thoracic column
   - AP supine
   - lateral
   - swimmer's view of upper column
3. Lumbar column and sacrum
   - AP supine
   - lateral-horizontal beam
   - AP pelvis

Cervical Region

In the cervical region, the most important projection is the lateral projection. Gehweiler has pointed out that at least two-thirds of significant pathology can be detected on this view (Table 3-2).[10] It is, therefore, mandatory that the surgeon and radiologist not rely solely on the lateral view to clear the cervical region in a trauma patient.[32]

From a practical standpoint, however, the presence of life-threatening injury outside of the vertebral column may dictate that the patient be taken immediately to surgery before a complete cervical series may be obtained. At our institution's trauma center, an initial diagnosis is made on the basis of a single lateral view, and the patient is kept in a hard cervical collar until such time as a complete cervical series may be obtained. Although some anesthesiologists may be reluctant to intubate such a patient, intubation by means of a nasotracheal tube may be accomplished rapidly without excessive neck motion and, even in the presence of severe fracture or dislocation, should not exacerbate an injury. It is in dealing with patients such as this that active consultation and cooperation among trauma surgeons, radiologists, neurosurgeons, and orthopedic surgeons is necessary. The treatment of life-threatening injuries precludes obtaining a complete series of radiographs.

At our institution all views are obtained routinely on a supine patient. In most instances, a portable x-ray unit is adequate for filming.

The lateral view is obtained by means of a horizontal beam with a grid cassette. A 40-inch focal film distance is utilized.

Table 3-2 Efficacy of Lateral Radiographs for Cervical Trauma

Injury	Demonstrable
Atlanto-occipital dislocation	+
Atlanto-axial dislocation	+
Atlas fractures	
• posterior arch	+
• anterior arch	+
• burst (Jefferson)	+/−
• lateral mass	−
• transverse process	−
Axis fractures	
• dens	+
• vertebral body	+
• vertebral arch ("hangman")	+
Lower cervical vertebral bodies	
• simple flexion	+
• burst	+
• uncinate process	−
Lower cervical vertebral arch	
• spinous process	+
• locked facets	+
• articular pillar	+/−
• lamina	+/−
• pedicle	−
• transverse process	−
Flexion sprain	+
Extension sprain	+
Flexion fracture–dislocation	+
Extension fracture–dislocation	+

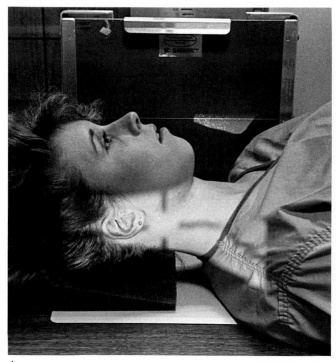
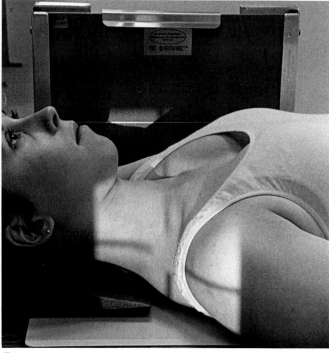

A   B

Figure 3-1 Lateral cervical view. **(A)** Standard horizontal beam technique. **(B)** "Swimmer's" view. In this instance, the patient's left arm is elevated.

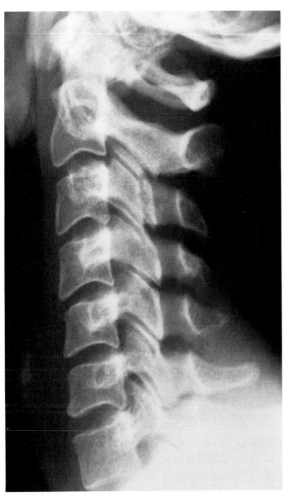

Figure 3-2 Normal lateral cervical radiograph. There is normal alignment of the anterior and posterior aspects of the vertebral bodies. The spinolaminar line is smooth and uninterrupted. The facet joints overlap in an orderly fashion (imbrication). The posterior vertebral body line is intact. The interspinous distance and interlaminar distance are uniform.

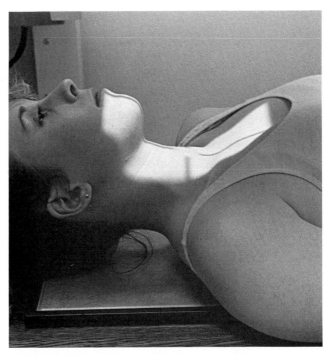

Figure 3-3 Standard AP cervical view.

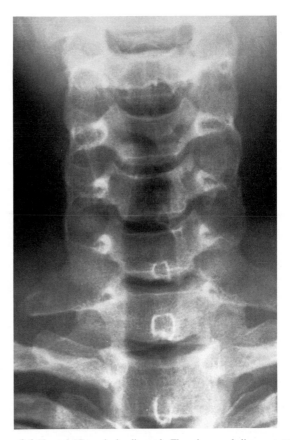

Figure 3-4 Normal AP cervical radiograph. There is normal alignment at the lateral margins. The pedicles are normally aligned and do not deviate more than 2 mm from level to level. The interspinous space is uniform. In this patient there are prominent transverse processes at C-7.

The film is placed adjacent to the patient's head as close to the shoulders as possible. Gentle traction is placed on the shoulders to make imaging of C-7 possible (Figs 3-1 and 3-2). Under no circumstances should traction be applied to the head.

In individuals with upper limb fractures, it may be impossible to place traction on the upper limbs. Additional views with the "swimmer's" technique may be necessary for complete imaging of the lower cervical region. Despite all these efforts, however, it still may be impossible to see C-6 and C-7 in muscular or obese patients with heavy shoulders. In these patients, lateral tomography may be necessary to clear this area. Nevertheless, in most instances the trauma oblique views will serve to clear the region.

After an adequate lateral radiograph has been obtained, the x-ray tube is placed in an upright position with 20° of cranial angulation of the central beam (Figs 3-3 and 3-4). The point of entry is at the cricoid cartilage (C-6). The film is placed beneath the patient's neck. This may be accomplished easily

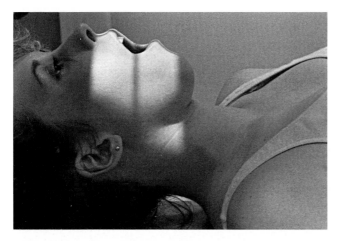

Figure 3-5 Technique for open-mouth atlanto-axial view. The mandible may be moved to blur out the shadows of the teeth if necessary.

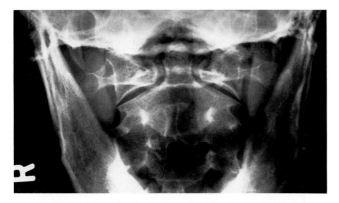

Figure 3-6 Normal atlanto-axial view. There is normal alignment between the lateral masses of C-1 and the lateral margin of the body of C-2. The spaces between the lateral masses of C-1 and the dens are uniform.

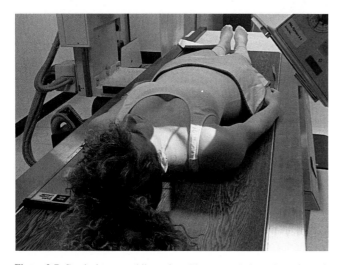

Figure 3-7 Cervical trauma oblique view. The x-ray tube is angled 35° to 40° off the horizontal with a 15° cranial tilt.

by placing the film under the backboard on which the patient is lying. Once again, a 40-inch focal film distance is used.[10]

The next view obtained is one of the atlanto-axial region with the patient's mouth open when possible (Figs 3-5 and 3-6); this view may be delayed until a patient is able to cooperate fully. To obtain this view, it may be necessary to remove the anterior portion of the cervical collar in which the patient has arrived. To prevent patient motion, sandbags should be placed at either side of the patient's head and secured with a generous amount of tape, or an assistant may hold the head. Angled views for demonstrating the arches of C-1 may also be necessary.[8]

One of the more interesting and valuable views is the trauma oblique projection. This view was developed independently at approximately the same time by Gehweiler[10] and Abel.[1] For this projection, the film is placed adjacent to the head and neck with the patient supine on the table. The x-ray tube is angled 30° to 40° off the horizontal (Fig 3-7).[1,10] With no additional tube angulation, the lower cervical region is not always adequately visualized because of the patient's shoulders (Fig 3-8). In 1983, this view was modified at our institution to include a 15° cranial tilt of the tube in addition to the off-horizontal tilt. The result of this additional angulation is that the cervicothoracic junction is demonstrable even in patients with heavy shoulders (Fig 3-9).

The resulting image from either of these techniques shows considerable distortion because of the angulation. Nevertheless, there is adequate demonstration of the vertebral bodies, the pedicles, the articular pillars, and the laminae.[1,10] In addition, the posterior arch of the atlas is clearly seen. Less well recognized is the fact that a pair of these radiographs essentially represents two views of the same region at 90° to each other. Thus the cardinal principle of radiographic diagnosis—to examine an injured part with two views at 90°—is preserved. A diagnosis in the lower cervical region, particularly on thick-necked individuals, can be made with confidence by means of a combination of the AP view and both trauma oblique views.

Before the patient leaves the emergency department or is discharged from the hospital, it is necessary to obtain an upright lateral view. This view is obtained because of the possibility of an occult flexion sprain (Figs 3-10 and 3-11).[10] This common injury is the result of posterior ligamentous damage. There are no accompanying fractures. The supine lateral radiograph may appear to be entirely normal, but an upright view will reveal acute kyphotic angulation, widening of the interspinous space, and facet widening due to the mechanical effect of the added weight of the patient's head.[10,15,16]

At our institution, active flexion and extension views are used on a limited basis. Other hospitals utilize these routinely. Bohrer conducted a study showing the value of the use of routine flexion and extension views, but other specialists believe that they are not necessary in every case. Flexion and extension views should be reserved for those individuals who have minor degrees of anterolisthesis or retrolisthesis. In most instances, the cause of this listhesis is degenerative disk dis-

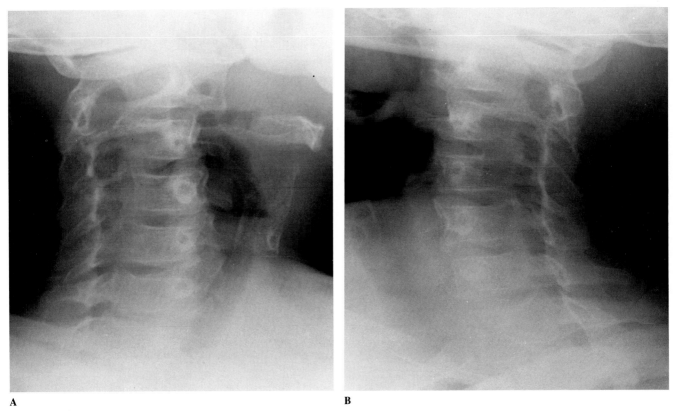

A   B

Figure 3-8 Normal trauma oblique films without additional tube angulation. Note the loss of definition at the cervicothoracic junction.

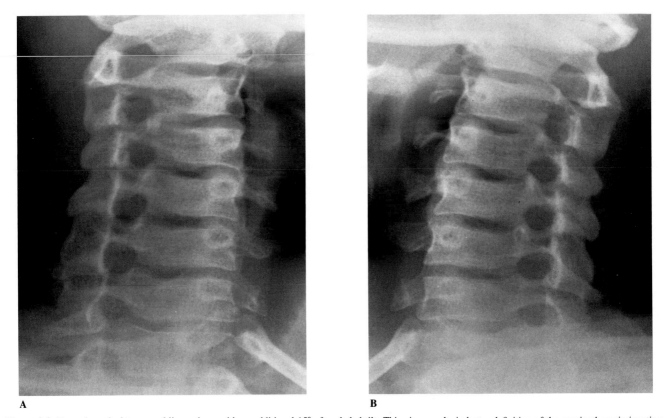

A   B

Figure 3-9 Normal cervical trauma oblique views with an additional 15° of cephalad tilt. This view results in better definition of the cervicothoracic junction. Compare with Fig 3-8.

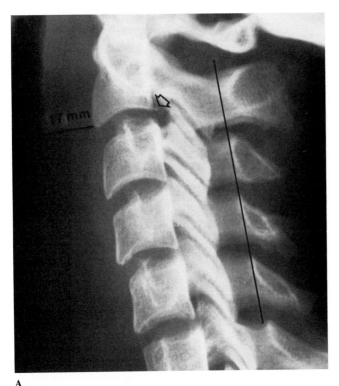
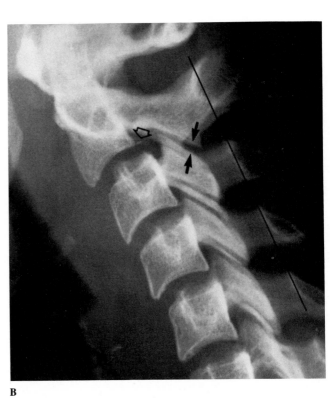

A   B

Figure 3-10 Flexion sprain. **(A)** Supine radiograph shows normal alignment of C-2 on C-3. There is, however, widening of the prevertebral soft tissue space to 17 mm (double arrow). A small avulsion fracture off the posteroinferior aspect of the body of C-2 is present (open arrow). The spinolaminar line is disrupted (straight line). **(B)** Lateral flexion film shows anterolisthesis of C-2 on C-3. There is widening of the facet joint of C2-3 (solid arrows). Note the disruption of the spinolaminar line. The avulsed fragment from the posteroinferior aspect of the body of C-2 again is shown (open arrow).

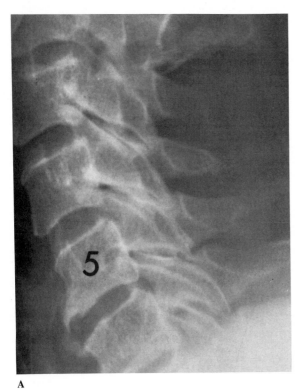
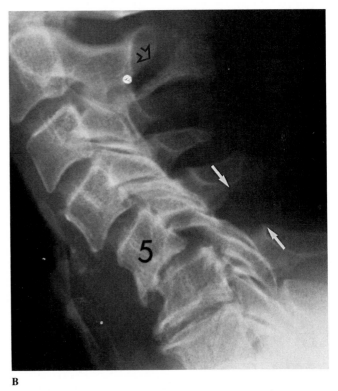

A   B

Figure 3-11 Flexion sprain. **(A)** Supine radiograph shows mild degenerative changes at the C-5 disk level. The alignment is otherwise normal. **(B)** An upright radiograph shows anterolisthesis of C-5 on C-6, narrowing of the C-5 disk space anteriorly, widening of the interspinous and interlaminar space of C5-6 (solid arrows), and marked widening of the facet joints. In addition, there is a fracture of the spinous process of C-2 (open arrow) that was not apparent on the supine radiograph. Flexion sprains of this variety will be missed unless an erect film is obtained before the patient is discharged.

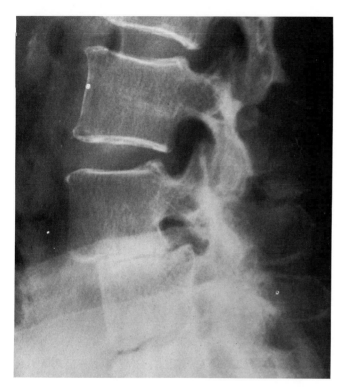

Figure 3-12 Anterolisthesis secondary to degenerative disk disease. Lateral lumbar radiograph shows anterolisthesis of L-4 on L-5. The disk spaces of L-4 and L-5 are narrow.

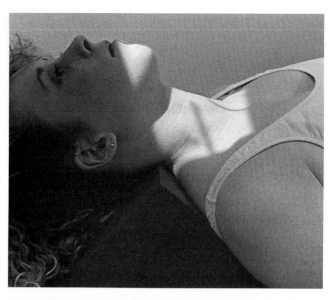

Figure 3-13 Vertebral arch ("pillar") view. The patient's neck is hyperextended. The central beam enters at C-6 at an angle of approximately 30° off the horizontal. This view would not be performed after acute trauma.

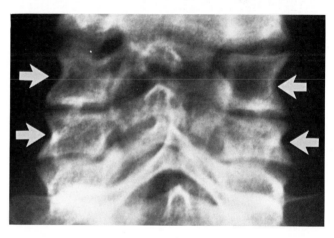

Figure 3-14 Vertebral arch view appearance. There is elongation and flattening of the articular pillars (arrows). This view is especially useful for defining these structures. This film was obtained from a standard AP view of a hyperextended patient with a C7-T1 dislocation.

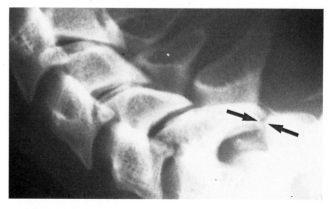

Figure 3-15 Bilateral jumped locked facets C7-T1. Lateral radiograph shows the point of locking (arrows). This patient was neurologically intact (same patient as in Fig 3-14).

ease at the same level (Fig 3-12). Under no circumstances should the patient's head be passively moved for this study. It is best to leave a cervical collar in place until the patient is able to cooperate fully.

Another view that is sometimes obtained is the vertebral arch view,[10] in which the tube is angled 30° from the horizontal in a caudal direction on a supine patient. The beam is centered on the suprasternal notch (Fig 3-13). This produces a distorted view of the cervical column and elongates the laminae and articular pillars (Fig 3-14). It has been found that the trauma oblique views combined with CT can provide sufficient clinical information; thus the vertebral arch view is rarely used.

In individuals with heavy shoulders or thick necks, it may be necessary to obtain a swimmer's view of the cervicothoracic junction. This requires that the patient have no injuries to one of the upper limbs. At our institution, trauma obliques are used more often than the swimmer's view to clear the cervicothoracic region.

In the cervical region, however, there are certain pitfalls and limitations. As previously mentioned, the adequate visualization of the cervicothoracic junction is sometimes difficult. Muscular or obese patients present special diagnostic problems. The failure to demonstrate adequately the cervicothoracic junction presents the hazard of missing an occult fracture or dislocation (Fig 3-15). Every effort should be made to obtain adequate views of this area, making use of all the views mentioned above.

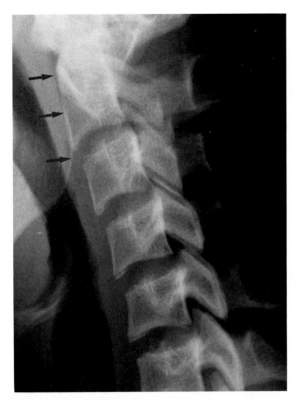

Figure 3-16 Normal cervical radiograph in a patient with cervical spasm. There is reversal of the normal lordosis. Note the position of the mandible, which is tucked in the "military" posture.

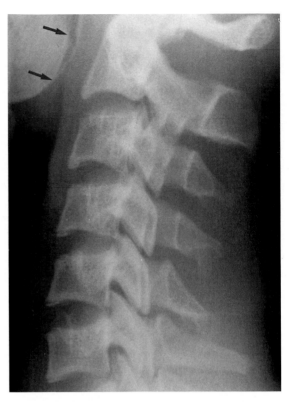

Figure 3-17 Same patient as in Fig. 3-16 in the upright position. The normal lordosis has been restored. Note the position of the mandible (arrows).

Another area of concern is the individual in whom there is straightening or reversal of the normal cervical lordosis. How can these patients, in whom the radiographic abnormality is purely due to position or muscle spasm, be differentiated from patients with true ligamentous injury? There are several helpful clues on the lateral radiograph that can provide the answer (Fig 3-16). First, if the abnormality is purely due to position, the angle of the mandible will be close to the cervical column ("military posture"). Second, there will be no disruption of the spinolaminar line; this indicates that no posterior ligamentous damage has occurred. Third, there will be no evidence of soft tissue abnormality in the prevertebral region. Fourth, in an older individual in whom there are minor degrees of anterolisthesis (see Fig 3-12), there will be evidence of degenerative disease at the level of the abnormality. The upright lateral view without a collar in an asymptomatic patient may solve the riddle (Fig 3-17). Nevertheless, it may be necessary to obtain flexion and extension views to determine whether a true alignment abnormality is present.

Thoracic and Lumbar Regions

The radiographic examination of the thoracic vertebral column may be accomplished with supine radiography. An AP view is obtained immediately after chest radiography (Figs 3-18 and 3-19), and then a horizontal beam lateral radiograph (Figs 3-20 and 3-21) is obtained. Because of the shoulders and arms, there is usually poor demonstration of the upper thoracic region, and it may be necessary to "log-roll" the patient into a lateral position to examine this area. A swimmer's view may be necessary as well.

Upper thoracic fractures are common in motorcyclists (Fig 3-22) and also in patients thrown from vehicles. These lesions are difficult to diagnose from chest radiographs, particularly in heavy individuals. It is therefore mandatory that thoracic radiographs be obtained in these patients.

In the lumbar region, AP supine and cross-table lateral radiographs should be adequate to diagnose most injuries (Figs 3-23 through 3-26). Sacral injuries are usually the result of pelvic fractures. An AP view of the pelvis is thus included as part of routine trauma screening series. It is usually not necessary to obtain oblique views of the lumbar vertebral column since frontal and lateral films are usually adequate.

The only pitfall in diagnosing an injury in the thoracic region is improper imaging of the upper thoracic column in a lateral position. It may be necessary to obtain lateral tomograms or CT scans of areas of suspected thoracic abnormality in the upper thoracic column (Fig 3-27). There are no pitfalls in diagnosing injuries in the lumbar region.

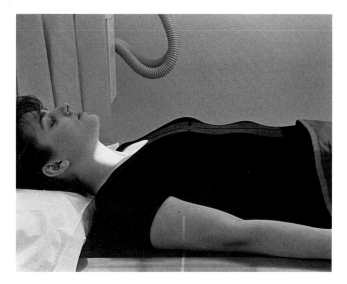

Figure 3-18 Normal thoracic column, AP view.

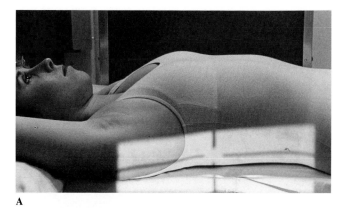

A

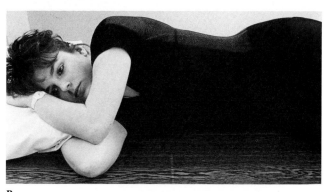

B

Figure 3-20 Lateral thoracic radiography. **(A)** Horizontal beam technique in a supine patient. **(B)** Vertical beam technique.

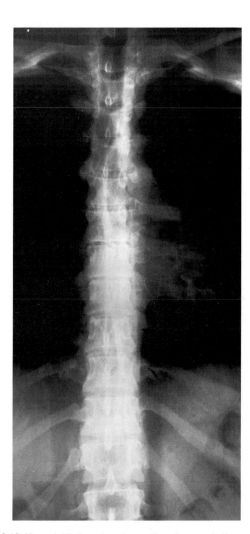

Figure 3-19 Normal AP thoracic column. There is normal alignment of the vertebral body margins, pedicles, and spinous processes. The interspinous space and the interpedicular distance are uniform. The paravertebral soft tissues are normal.

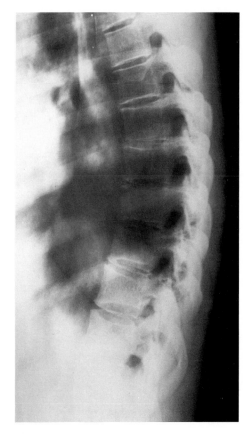

Figure 3-21 Normal thoracic column. Lateral view shows normal alignment with gentle kyphosis. The disk margins are uniform.

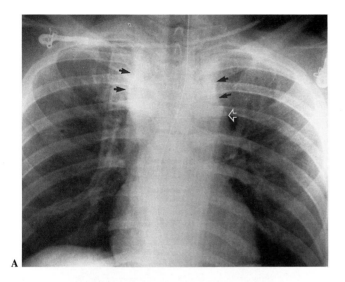

A

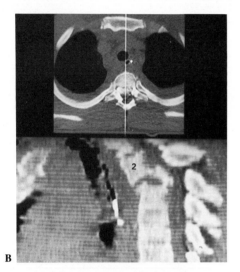

B

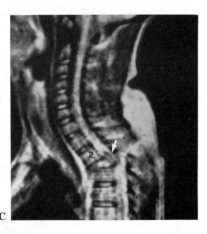

C

Figure 3-22 Occult thoracic injury in a motorcyclist. **(A)** Supine chest radiograph shows widening of the superior mediastinum (solid arrows). The aortic shadow (open arrow) is sharply defined. This indicates posterior mediastinal widening. **(B)** CT scan with sagittal reconstruction shows fracture-dislocation of T2-3. **(C)** MRI examination ($T_R = 2.1$, $T_E = 35$) shows the full extent of injury with complete transection of the spinal cord by a bone fragment from T-3 (arrow). *Source:* Reprinted with permission from ''Thoracic Fractures and Dislocations in Motorcyclists'' by RH Daffner et al in *Skeletal Radiology* (1987;16:280–284), Copyright © 1987, Springer-Verlag.

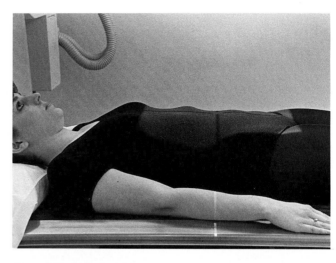

Figure 3-23 AP lumbar view.

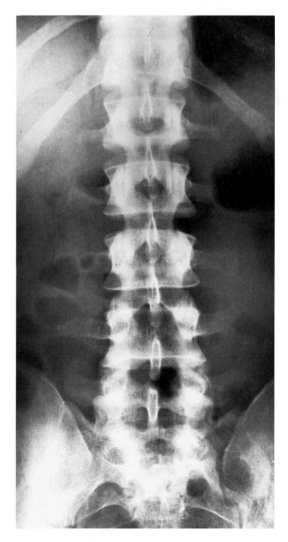

Figure 3-24 AP view of a normal lumbar column. There is normal alignment of the vertebral bodies, transverse processes, and pedicles. The interspinous spaces are uniform, as are the interpedicular distances.

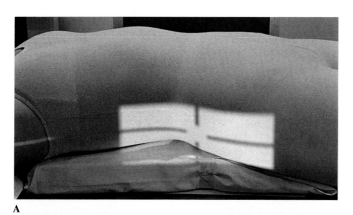

A

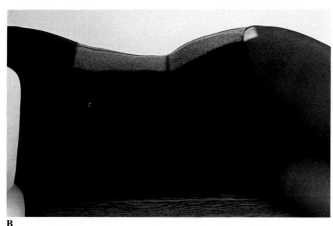

B

Figure 3-25 Lateral lumbar radiography. **(A)** Horizontal beam technique. **(B)** Vertical beam technique.

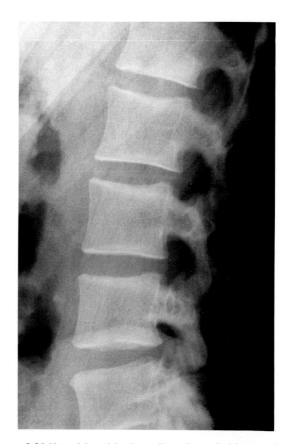

Figure 3-26 Normal lateral lumbar radiograph, vertical beam technique. There is normal alignment of the vertebral bodies. The posterior vertebral body lines are either single or bifid at the level of the nutrient canal. The disk spaces are uniform. This view is not satisfactory for assessing the interspinous distance.

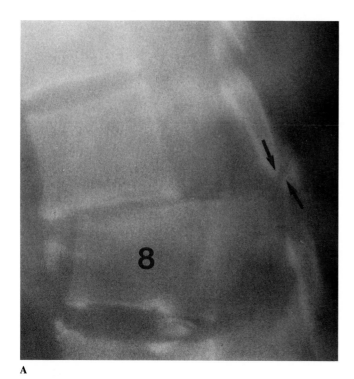

A

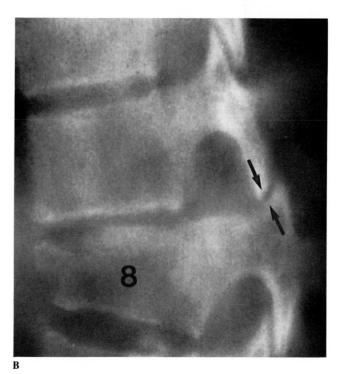

B

Figure 3-27 Thoracic fracture–dislocation with bilateral facet locking. Lateral tomograms show the fracture of the body of T-8 with locking of the facets of T-7 and T-8 (arrows).

COMPUTED TOMOGRAPHY

The development of CT in the early 1970s revolutionized the practice of diagnostic radiology. For the first time it was possible to obtain cross-sectional images of areas hitherto unseen by noninvasive diagnostic methods. It soon became apparent that one of the prime diagnostic uses for CT would be for the evaluation of patients with vertebral trauma.[2,4,5,9,11,12,14,21,24,26,29,30,33,35]

The principles of CT are well known and need not be discussed here. The study is easy to perform. The patient must lie in a supine position and not move. To obtain an adequate study in an acutely injured patient, it may be necessary to induce immobility pharmacologically. There is no standard number of images obtained. In our institution, the standard procedure is to determine the levels for examination from plain films and from the CT scout view. Imaging is then performed from one complete vertebral level above to one complete vertebral level below the area of suspected injury. Sections are obtained contiguously at 4- to 5-mm intervals, depending on the machine used. Sections are not overlapped. Filming is performed with both bone and soft tissue windows (Fig 3-28). Intravenous contrast enhancement is not required.

Scout views are obtained to determine the level of the scan. In the cervical region, they are performed in the lateral position; in the thoracic region, in the AP position; and in the lumbar region, either in the AP or lateral position. A full-size view is obtained with and without level annotations.

Computed tomography provides an additional plane of examination with additional information about the extent of injury.[5,29,30,33,35] It is the best method for determining the presence and degree of canal encroachment (Fig 3-29) or intervertebral foramen encroachment (Fig 3-30). It is also useful for demonstrating fractures of the laminae, pedicles (Figs 3-31 and 3-32), and articular pillars, particularly those associated with perched or locked facets[33,35] where the images of both facets of the joint are present (Fig 3-33). The ability to perform sagittal and coronal reconstructions with CT is an additional benefit.

In many institutions, CT is combined with myelography using a water-soluble contrast medium to evaluate traumatic encroachment of the subarachnoid space and spinal cord by bone fragments or herniated intervertebral disk fragments (Figs 3-34 and 3-35). CT with myelography is also useful for studying cervical nerve root avulsions[28] (Fig 3-36) and post-traumatic cystic myelopathy.[31] In many institutions, CT with myelography is performed because MRI is not available or, if it is available, the patient is too unstable for the study to be done.

Software programs for CT are now available that will allow three-dimensional (3D) reconstruction (Fig 3-37).[34] Clinicians find this program to be more useful in determining the spatial relationships of bone fragments. The true value of 3D reconstruction remains to be determined.

There are pitfalls and limitations to the use of CT.[19,29,30] These may be divided into patient-related causes and technical pitfalls. Patient-related pitfalls result from motion, patient

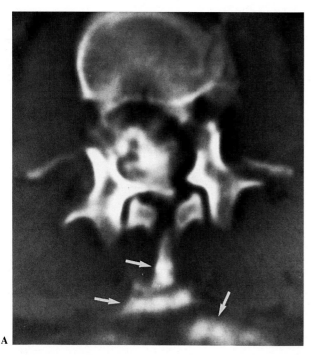

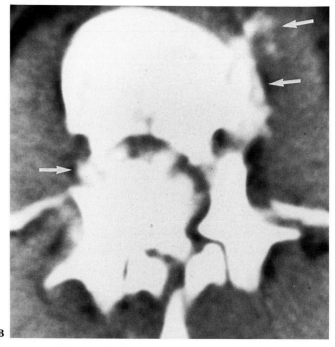

Figure 3-28 Severely comminuted lumbar fracture with extravasation of intrathecal contrast medium. **(A)** CT at bone window shows the severely comminuted fracture of the vertebra. Intrathecal contrast medium is extravasated (arrows). **(B)** Soft tissue window shows further extravasation anteriorly into the paraspinal soft tissues (arrows). These areas of extravasation were not as easily identifiable on the bone window image (same patient as in Fig 3-60).

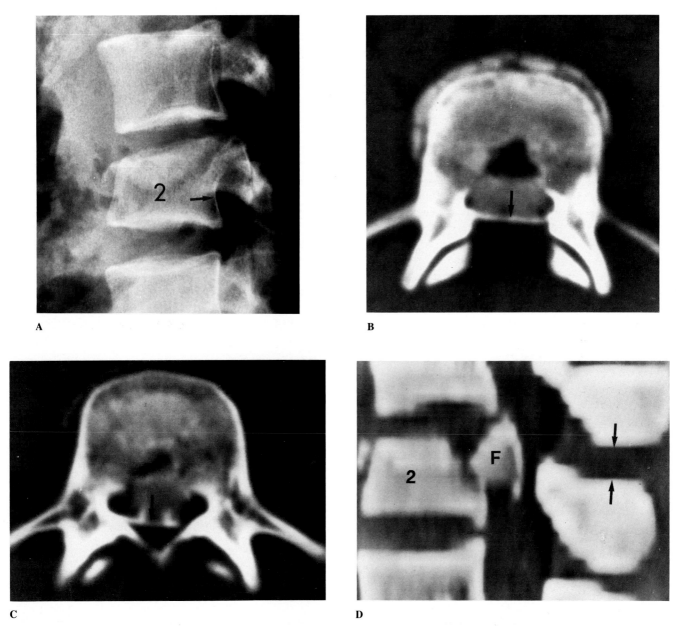

Figure 3-29 Burst fracture of L-2. **(A)** Lateral radiograph shows compression of the body of L-2. Note the interruption of the posterior vertebral body line (arrow). This indicates retropulsion of a fracture fragment. **(B and C)** CT scan shows fractures of the body anteriorly and retropulsion of a central bony fragment to encroach on the vertebral canal (arrows). **(D)** Sagittal reconstruction of CT images shows the large free fragment (F) that has been displaced into the vertebral canal. Note the widening of the interspinous space (arrows).

size, and artifacts from metallic implants. Motion on the study results in blurred images and the possibility of a missed diagnosis. The patient's weight is also a serious consideration. Most CT machines have a patient weight limit of 300 pounds because the table must project into the gantry for the examination. Another patient-related problem relates to previous spinal surgery with implantation of internal fixation rods. In these individuals, the metallic rods cause serious artifacts that compromise the radiographic image.

There are three technical pitfalls that may result in incomplete information being obtained from the radiograph. These are the averaging effect, poor level calibration, and fractures in the plane of the scan. Partial volume-averaging effect is a well-known pitfall in CT. Normally, CT gives an image that represents an average of the radiographic densities of all structures contained within that section of tissue. Any normal structure or abnormality that is not completely located within the plane of scan may be distorted or totally discarded from the

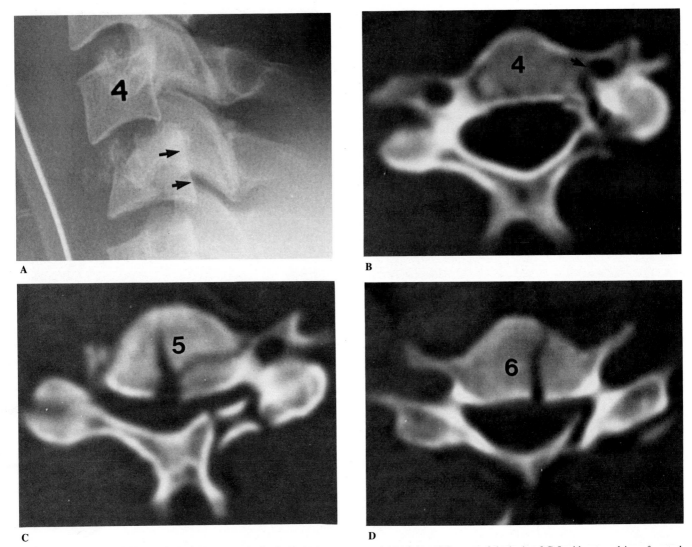

A   **B**

C   **D**

Figure 3-30 Cervical burst fracture–dislocation. **(A)** Lateral radiograph shows severely comminuted fracture of the body of C-5 with retropulsion of central fragment to encroach on the vertebral canal (arrows). There is flattening of the body of C-6 as well. **(B)** CT scan shows a fracture through the inferior articular pillar of C-4 with encroachment of the intervertebral foramen on the left (arrow). This fracture was unsuspected clinically. **(C)** CT section through C-5 shows the burst fracture of the body C-5 with severe canal compromise. There are fractures through the lamina on the left. **(D)** CT section through C-6 shows fracture of the body as well as fracture through the lamina on the left. This fracture, along with that of C-4, was unsuspected on the basis of the lateral radiograph. This case illustrates the utility of CT in identifying additional unsuspected fractures.

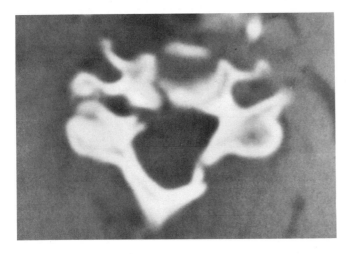

Figure 3-31 CT scan showing severely comminuted fractures of a cervical vertebra involving the body, pedicle on the right, and lamina on the left. Note the distortion of the vertebral canal.

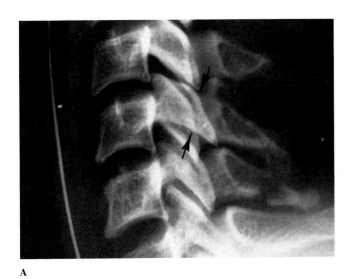

A

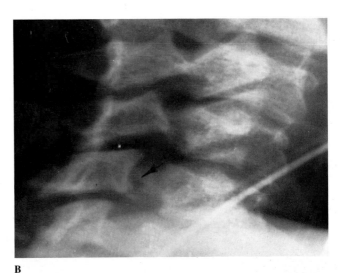

B

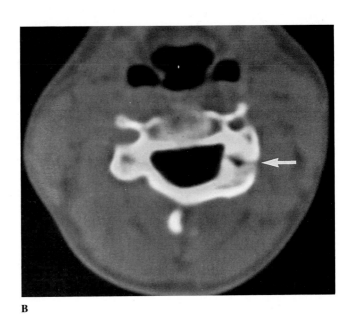

FLOATING
PILLAR

C

Figure 3-32 Cervical fractures with floating articular pillar. (**A**) Lateral radiograph shows duplication of the pillar images of C-5 (arrows). All the other levels show superimposed pillar images. (**B**) Trauma oblique view shows fracture through the pedicle of C-5 on the right side (arrow). (**C**) CT scan shows asymmetry of the pillars with a floating pillar on the right (arrow). This case illustrates the ability of CT to elucidate confusing plain film radiographic images.

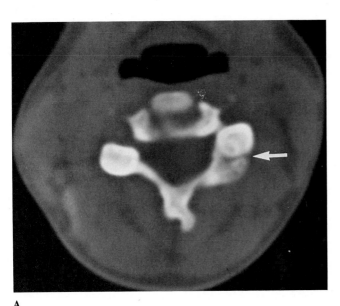

A

B

Figure 3-33 Locked facets, CT appearance. (**A and B**) CT sections show duplication of facet images on the left (arrows) at the point of locking (same patient as in Fig 4-24).

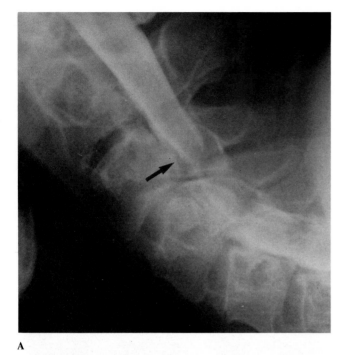

A

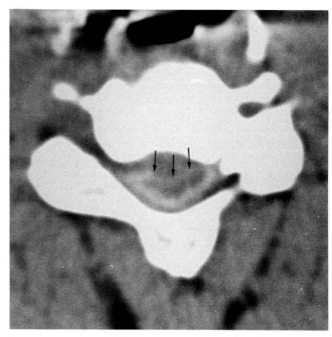

B

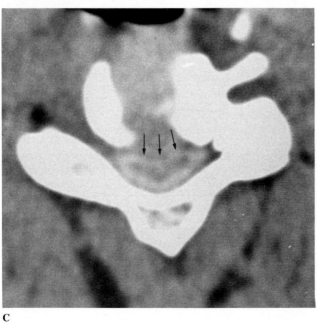

C

Figure 3-34 Posttraumatic herniated intervertebral disk space C3-4 in a patient with a burst fracture of C-3. (A) Myelogram shows bone fragment encroaching on the vertebral canal (arrow). Note the attenuation of the contrast-filled subarachnoid space. (B and C) CT with myelography immediately after (A) shows herniated disk material encroaching on the subarachnoid space (arrows). (B, just above disk level; C, at disk level.)

final image (Fig 3-38). In most instances, a fracture will be seen on more than one cross-section. It is possible, however, particularly in dealing with thin structures, such as the laminae or posterior arch of C-1, that an abnormality is seen on one view only (Fig 3-39). Furthermore, where there is normal overlap of structures from adjacent vertebrae there will be apparent lines of interruption in the bony shadow (Fig 3-40); these should not be misinterpreted as fractures.

In some machines, a discrepancy in annotation on the scout film may result in erroneous information being obtained about the level of injury. This generally does not present a significant problem because plain film examination should determine the levels of fracture.

Fractures that are oriented in a horizontal plane may not always be demonstrated by CT. This occurs most commonly with fractures of the dens or body of C-2 (Fig 3-41). To overcome this pitfall, it may be necessary to tilt the gantry to bring the fracture out of the plane of the scan. In some cases, it may be necessary to resort to conventional tomography to define further the extent of the fracture.

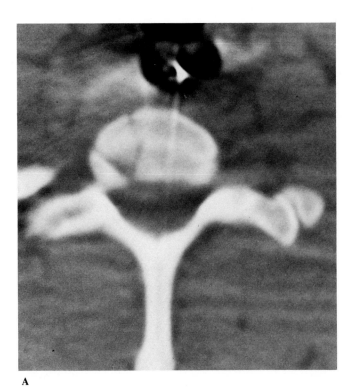

A

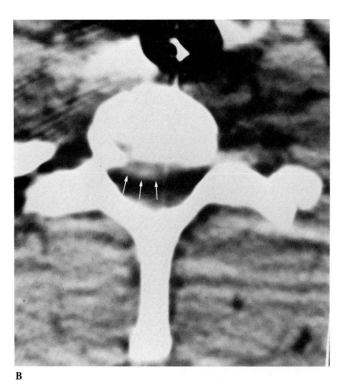

B

Figure 3-35 Posttraumatic herniated intervertebral disk in a patient with a fracture of C-6. **(A)** CT scan at bone window shows fractures of the body of C-6 on the right. **(B)** Soft tissue window view at the same level shows herniated disk material (arrows).

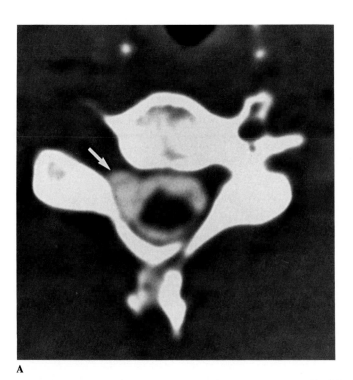

A

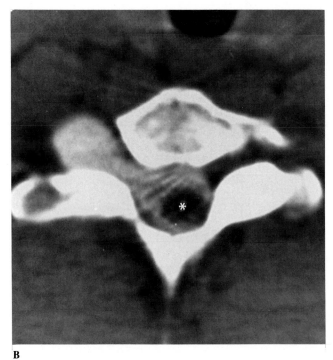

B

Figure 3-36 Cervical nerve root avulsion as a result of C6-7 fractures. **(A)** CT myelogram shows extravasated contrast along the root sheath (arrow) at the neural foramen. Note the fractured lamina on the left. **(B)** One level lower. The extravasated contrast follows the nerve sheath further laterally. Note the cord (*) displaced toward the left (same patient as in Fig 3-61).

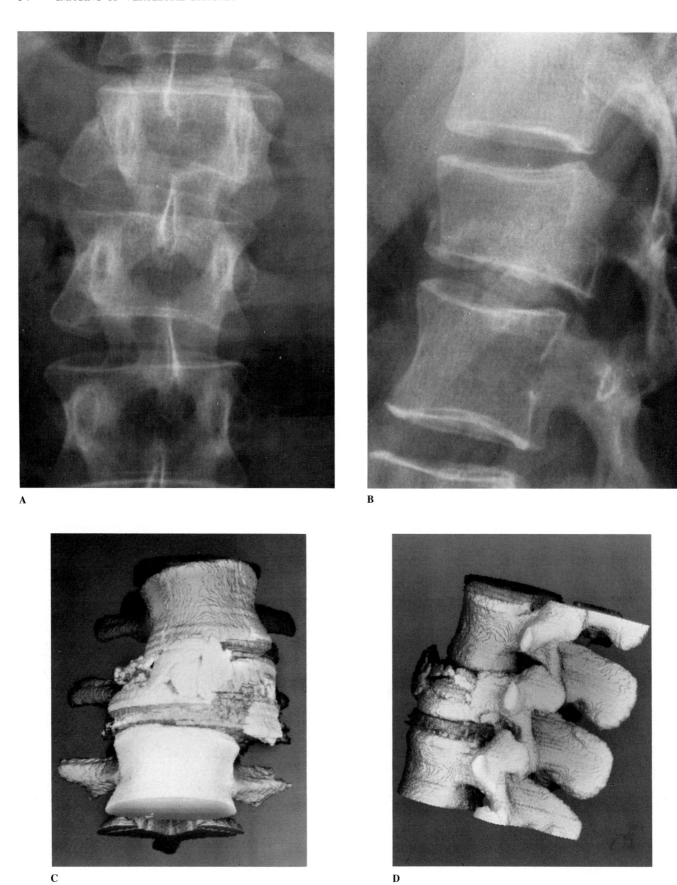

Figure 3-37 Use of 3-dimensional (3D) reconstruction. **(A)** Frontal and **(B)** lateral radiographs show a burst fracture of L-1. **(C)** Frontal and **(D)** lateral 3D reconstructions of a similar injury show the spatial relationships of the bone fragments.

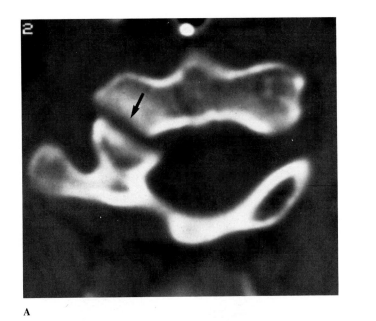

A

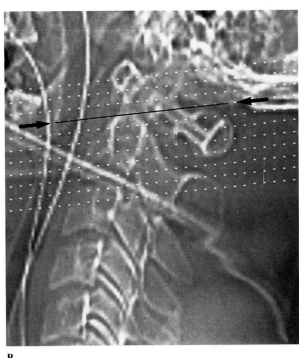

B

Figure 3-38 Partial volume effect. **(A)** CT scan through C-2 shows apparent fracture through the pedicle on the right (arrow). This is due to partial volume effect in a patient whose head was tilted in the gantry. **(B)** The scout view shows a reverse angle to the plane of the scan in an attempt to avoid artifacts from dental fillings. The arrows illustrate the slice shown in **A**.

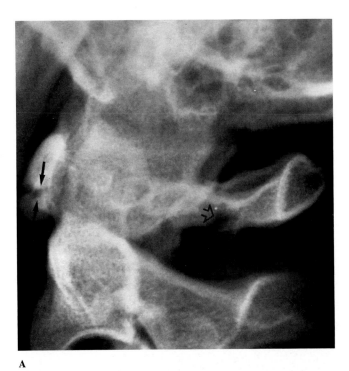

A

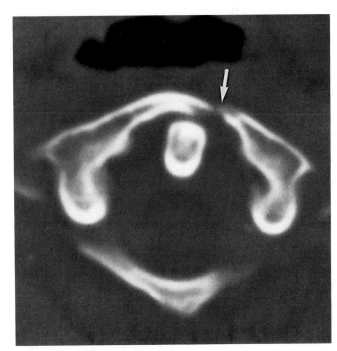

B

Figure 3-39 Jefferson fracture of C-1. **(A)** Lateral radiograph shows horizontal fracture through the anterior arch of C-1 (solid arrows) as well as a fracture of the posterior arch (open arrow). **(B)** CT section shows the anterior arch fracture on this view only (arrow).

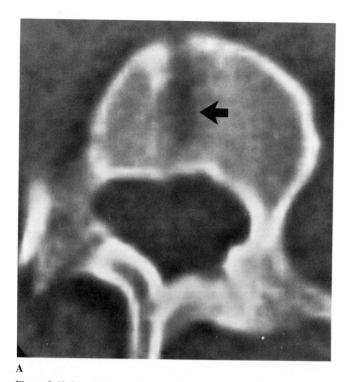

A

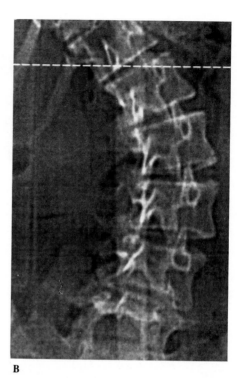

B

Figure 3-40 Pseudofracture due to partial volume effect in a patient with scoliosis. **(A)** CT section shows apparent fracture through the vertebral body (arrow). **(B)** Digital scout view image shows a severe levorotoscoliosis. The image obtained is actually a composite of T-12 and L-1. *Source:* Reprinted with permission from "Spinal Deformities and Pseudofractures" by MI Boechat in *American Journal of Roentgenology* (1987;148:97–98), Copyright © 1987, American Roentgen Ray Society.

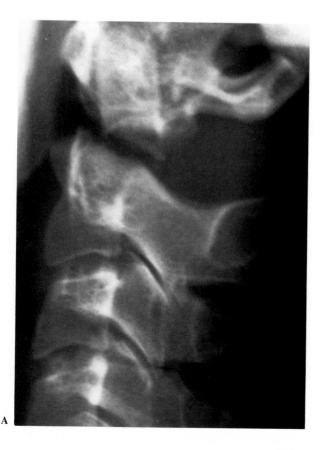

A

Figure 3-41 Dens fracture. **(A)** Lateral radiograph shows a fracture at the base of the dens with retrolisthesis of the dens and C-1. **(B)** CT scan through the base of the dens does not show the fracture. In this case, the fracture is oriented in the same plane as the CT scan.

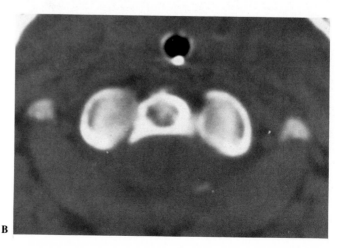

B

CONVENTIONAL POLYDIRECTIONAL TOMOGRAPHY

The use of CT has practically eliminated the use of conventional tomography for the diagnosis of vertebral injuries. Nevertheless, there still is a use for this older modality.[3,10,15,16,18,22] Most hospitals are now equipped with complex-motion (polydirectional) tomographic units (PT), but even simple linear tomography may be used when needed.

Conventional tomography may be used to supplement plain film and CT examinations. This is considered by many radiologists to be the best method for evaluating the axis to differentiate between a Mach band and dens fracture at C-2 (Figs 3-42 and 3-43). Other uses are for evaluation of articular

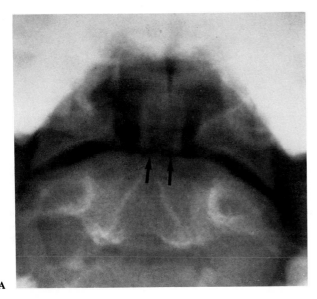

A

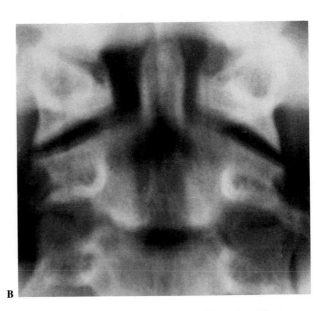

B

Figure 3-42 Mach band at C-2. **(A)** There is a horizontal lucency across the base of the dens on this plain film (arrows) due to Mach band formation. **(B)** Tomogram through the area shows no evidence of fracture.

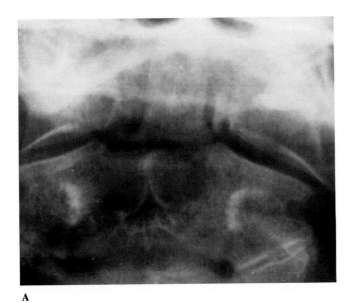

A

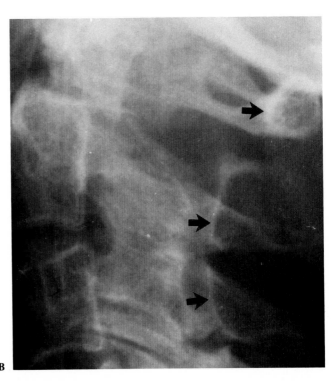

B

Figure 3-43 Dens fracture. **(A)** Open-mouth, atlanto-axial view shows a lucent line across the base of the dens. There is also atlanto-axial offset toward the left. **(B)** The lateral view shows posterior displacement of the dens and C-1 in relation to C-2. Note the disruption of the spinolaminar line (arrows).

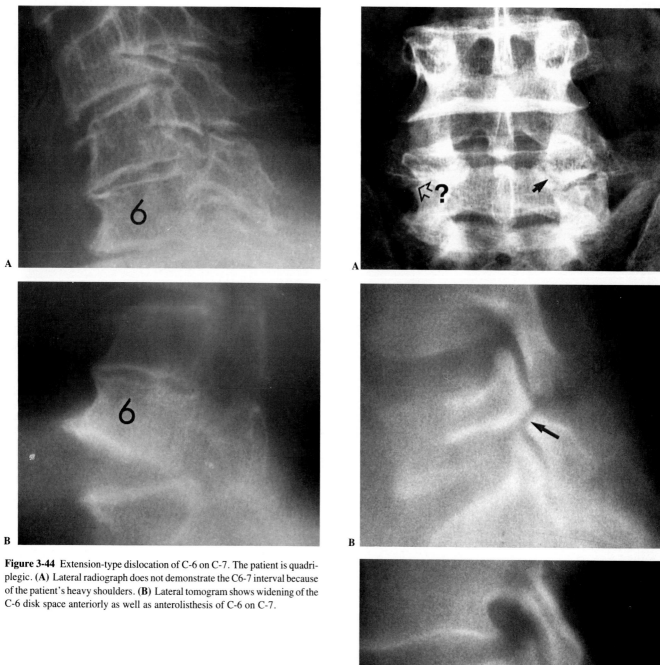

Figure 3-44 Extension-type dislocation of C-6 on C-7. The patient is quadriplegic. (**A**) Lateral radiograph does not demonstrate the C6-7 interval because of the patient's heavy shoulders. (**B**) Lateral tomogram shows widening of the C-6 disk space anteriorly as well as anterolisthesis of C-6 on C-7.

pillars and occasionally to rule out injury to the cervicothoracic junction in individuals with thick necks or shoulders where plain film evaluation is not satisfactory (Fig 3-44). Conventional tomography is also useful in the lower lumbar region for evaluating the pars interarticularis for spondylolysis. It is not necessary to perform a dual set of oblique tomograms. Simple lateral tomography will pass through both sides of the pars, and an abnormality, if present, will be clearly seen (Fig 3-45).

The only serious pitfall of conventional tomography is the formation of phantom images. This phenomenon is caused by the image of a structure out of the plane of focus being projected across the area of interest (Fig 3-46).

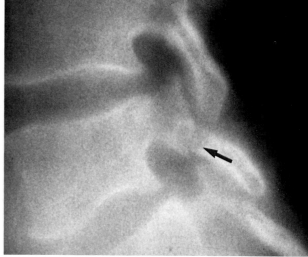

Figure 3-45 Conventional tomography in a patient with suspected bilateral pars interarticularis defect. (**A**) Frontal radiograph shows a lucency across the pars interarticularis of L-5 on the left (solid arrow). There is a question of a similar pars defect on the right (open arrow). (**B and C**) Lateral tomograms show bilateral pars interarticularis defects (arrows).

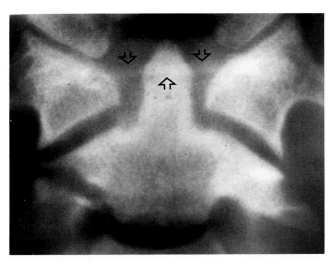

Figure 3-46 Phantom images. Horizontal line (open arrows) in the transverse plane across the dens and adjacent joint space represents the phantom image of the anterior arch of the atlas projected over the dens.

MAGNETIC RESONANCE IMAGING

The development of CT was a revolutionary step in diagnostic imaging and is believed to have been the most significant advance in radiology since the discovery of the roentgen ray. Less than 10 years after its development, the radiologic world would be excited by the advent of MRI. One of the first areas to be evaluated by this modality was the vertebral column.

Although initial interest in most vertebral studies related to the diagnosis of disk disease, it soon became apparent that MRI would be useful for evaluating patients who had suffered vertebral trauma.[6,13,17,20,23] By altering the technical factors of echo time and recovery time, it was demonstrated that sagittal images could be obtained rapidly and give osseous positional detail (Fig 3-47) as well as demonstrate the state of disk hydration and the interface between cerebrospinal fluid (CSF) and extradural space. Exact scanning parameters will vary from institute to institute and depend on the type of machine used, the magnet strength, the type of coil used, and the patient's condition.

All of the MR images in this book were made on a Siemens Magnetom 0.5 tesla (T) operated at 0.35 to 0.5 T. The usual vertebral column examination consists of a short spin-echo sequence with an echo time (T_E) of 15 to 90 msec and a recovery or repetition time (T_R) of 300 to 600 msec in the sagittal plane. This provides rapid anatomic orientation and detail. In our institution, T_1 parameters of 15 to 35 msec T_E and 300 to 500 msec T_R with four repetitions and 5-mm slice thickness are used. A special surface coil is used for the spine; these vary according to the manufacturer. Five slices within approximately 9 minutes can thus be produced. This technique is excellent for demonstrating normal vertebral alignment and bony relationships to the spinal cord, particularly in

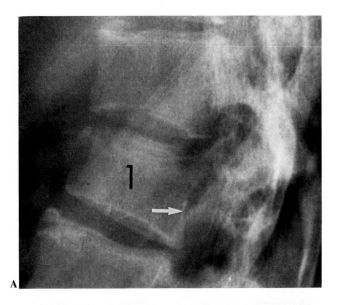

A

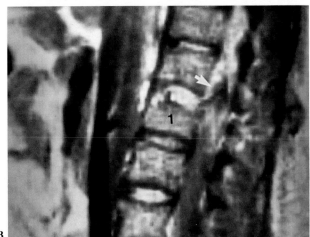

B

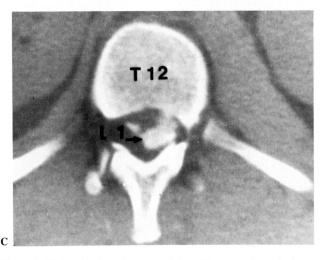

C

Figure 3-47 Complex burst fracture of L-1. **(A)** Lateral radiograph shows compression of the bodies of L-1 superiorly and of the inferior aspect of T-12. The superior aspect of the posterior vertebral body line (arrow) is absent, indicating a displaced fragment. **(B)** MRI examination (T_R = 2.1, T_E = 35) shows the displaced bone fragment within the vertebral canal (arrow). **(C)** CT examination through the inferior aspect of T-12 shows the fragment within the canal.

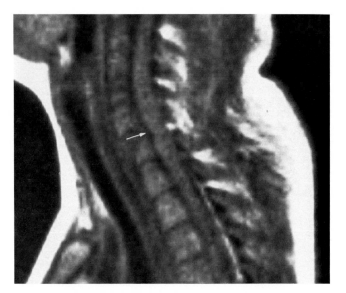

Figure 3-48 MRI examination in a patient with a C-6 burst fracture. This T_1-weighted image ($T_R = 0.3$, $T_E = 17$) shows encroachment of the subarachnoid space (arrow). There is no bony detail on this study. Compare with Fig 3-51.

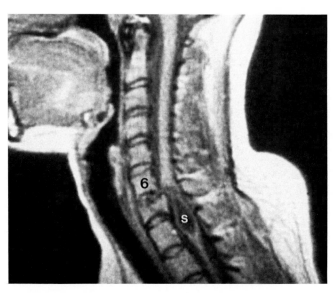

Figure 3-49 Posttraumatic syringomyelia. This patient suffered a burst fracture of C-7. MRI examination ($T_R = 0.5$, $T_E = 35$) performed 6 months after injury shows a localized low-signal area within the spinal cord representing a syrinx (s).

spinal cord compression[6,13,17,20,23] (Fig 3-48) and also is useful for demonstrating syringomyelia (Fig 3-49) and bone marrow replacement in malignant disease (Fig 3-50).[7]

A second, longer spin-echo sequence with a T_E of 35 to 100 msec and a T_R of 2000 to 3000 msec at T_2 and proton density weighting allows the evaluation of disk hydration and of the interface of the CSF and the extradural space. In this sequence, the signal intensity of the CSF is higher than surrounding structures; this is useful in evaluating patients with suspected extradural compression from bone fragments (Fig 3-51). This sequence is also obtained in the sagittal plane. Only one acquisition is made with these parameters, which results in approximately nine slices at a 7-mm interval. This sequence, too, takes approximately 9 minutes. A third sequence done in the transverse plane utilizes 35 to 70 msec T_E and 2100 msec T_R.[6,13,17,20,23] This provides high signal in the CSF and is useful for evaluation of the intervertebral disks. This modality is generally not used for evaluation of trauma patients.

''Fast scans'' have been advocated for demonstrating injuries in the axial (transverse) plane. These studies are performed using high field strength magnets (1.5 T) at short ($T_E = 0.11$, $T_R = 0.4$–1.5) sequences. Under these conditions, the CSF has high signal and thus helps to outline the spinal cord.

Table 3-3 summarizes scanning parameters.

Surface coils 13 to 22 cm long recessed within the patient couch are now being used. The body coil is used to transmit the signal, and surface coils are used to receive the signal. The surface coils result in improved images and decreased signal-to-noise ratio (Figs 3-52 and 3-53).

The short and long sagittal sequences are used in most trauma patients who are considered stable enough to be exam-

ined by MRI. If only one set of images can be obtained, the long sequence, which takes the same amount of time as the short sequence, is preferred. Sagittal images are primarily relied upon, and these are used to determine the degree of encroachment of the subarachnoid space and spinal cord (Figs 3-54 and 3-55). In our institution, MRI has now resulted in the nearly complete abandonment of myelography in trauma patients.

As mentioned above, MRI is useful in determining the relationship of bony fragments that may have been displaced into the vertebral canal to the spinal cord (Figs 3-48 and 3-51). MRI also can show the full extent of injury, especially the soft tissue damage associated with the injury (Figs 3-54 and 3-55). Recently, there has been interest in demonstration of acute spinal cord injury.[6,17,20] In addition to transection of the spinal cord, it is now possible to diagnose and differentiate spinal cord hemorrhage and edema.[6,17,20] An acutely traumatized spinal cord expands to fill the vertebral canal with concomitant obliteration of epidural fat, as a result of either hemorrhage or edema.[6,13,17,20] Acute spinal cord hemorrhage produces decreased signal intensity on T_2-weighted images obtained within 24 hours of injury.[13,20] Paraspinal hemorrhage, on the other hand, has high signal with T_2-weighting within and after 24 hours (Fig 3-51). Edema and contusion of the cord produce high signal intensity on T_2-weighted images (Figs 3-56 and 3-57).[6,13,20] Kulkarni and colleagues have shown that there is direct correlation between the appearance of the injured spinal cord on MRI and recovery of neurologic function. They found that those patients with cord edema or contusion recovered significant function, whereas those with hemorrhage did not (Figs 3-51 and 3-56).[20]

Magnetic resonance imaging is especially useful for assessing the vertebral anatomy and alignment in the cervicothoracic

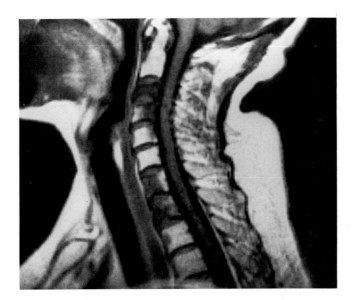

Figure 3-50 Metastases. Multiple metastatic lesions manifest as areas of low signal within the vertebral column. There is compression of C-3 with involvement of the subarachnoid space ($T_R = 0.3$, $T_E = 17$).

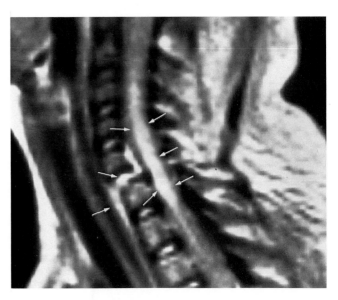

Figure 3-51 Burst fracture of C-6, canal encroachment, and cord hemorrhage. This T_2-weighted image of the same patient as in Fig 3-48 shows areas of hemorrhage that manifest as high signal (increased brightness) involving the spinal cord, epidural space, disk space, and prevertebral spaces (arrows). The T_2-weighted image is more suitable for identification of tissue characteristics ($T_R = 2.1$, $T_E = 35$).

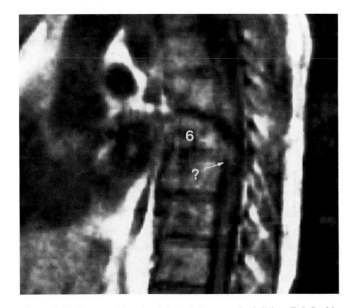

Figure 3-52 Suspected herniated thoracic intervertebral disk at T-6. In this patient, for whom a surface coil was not used, the detail at the T-6 disk level is poor. Irregularity at that level (arrow) cannot be differentiated from noise seen elsewhere in the study ($T_R = 0.3$, $T_E = 17$). Compare with Fig 3-53.

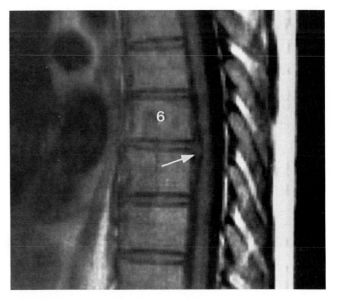

Figure 3-53 Same patient as in Fig 3-52. This study was made with a surface coil and clearly shows a herniated intervertebral disk at T-6 (arrow). Note the improved detail and signal-to-noise ratio ($T_R = 0.3$, $T_E = 17$).

Table 3-3 Common Vertebral MRI Scanning Parameters*

Sequence	T_E (msec)	T_R (msec)	No. of Measurements	No. of Slices	Slice Thickness (mm)	Time (min)
T1-weighting	15–35	300–500	4	5	5	9
T2-weighting	35–100	2000–3000	1	9	7	9
"Fast scan"†	11	0.4	4	5	7	5

*1988 figures, Siemens Magnetom, field strength 0.35–1.5 tesla.
†1.5 tesla or higher.

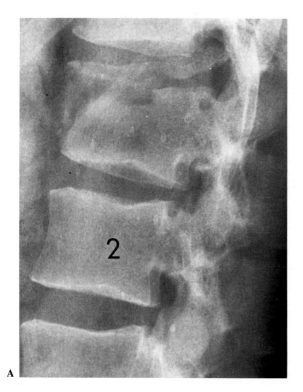

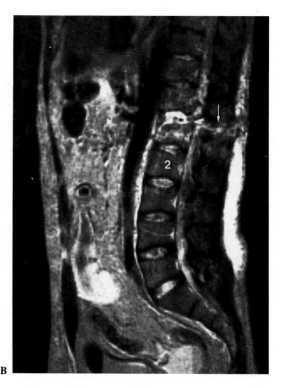

Figure 3-54 Burst fracture of L-1. **(A)** Lateral radiograph shows disruption of L-1 extending into the vertebral canal. **(B)** MRI examination ($T_R = 2.1$, $T_E = 35$) shows total disruption of L-1. High signal about the T-12 disk space, body of L-1, and posterior vertebral soft tissues indicate hemorrhage. Note the extent of injury posteriorly (arrow).

area (Fig 3-55). This area is nearly impossible to demonstrate because of the overlying shoulders. MRI can clearly show abnormalities in this region that would have necessitated lateral tomography in the past. Finally, MRI is extremely beneficial in the diagnosis of posttraumatic spinal cord cysts or syringomyelia (Fig 3-49). Again, MRI has superseded myelography for this purpose at our institution.

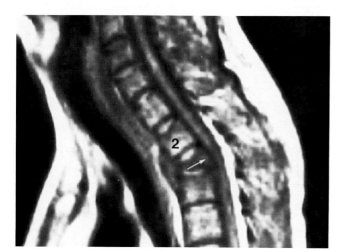

Figure 3-55 Fracture-dislocation of T-3 on T-4. MRI shows the fracture fragment of T-3 encroaching on the spinal cord (arrow). Lateral tomography would have been necessary to show the skeletal injury ($T_R = 0.5$, $T_E = 35$).

Magnetic resonance imaging has several advantages over CT for spinal imaging. These include the exploitation of inherent tissue contrast that can be manipulated by changing T_E and T_R; identification of vascular structures because of flow-produced characteristic signals; direct imaging in sagittal, coronal, transverse, axial, and occasionally para-axial planes; the absence of bone artifact; and the ability to image obese patients without signal loss.[6,7,13,17] High-strength MRI units (1.5 T) can show the loss of gray-white matter interface after injury.[6,20] Among the disadvantages of MRI for imaging trauma patients are that detailed skeletal anatomy is less than that obtained with CT, that patients requiring paramagnetic life support equipment cannot be imaged, and that patients with cervical halos cannot be studied. Improvements in monitoring equipment and nonmagnetic halo material should eliminate these problems in the future.[23]

MYELOGRAPHY

Myelography was used extensively in the past to determine the presence of blockage of flow of CSF by bone fragments in the vertebral canal or from meningeal injury (Figs 3-58 and 3-59). The use of MRI in many institutions has superseded myelography for this purpose. In those hospitals where MRI is unavailable, myelography still may be useful in this regard. In addition to diagnosing blockage of the flow of CSF, myelogra-

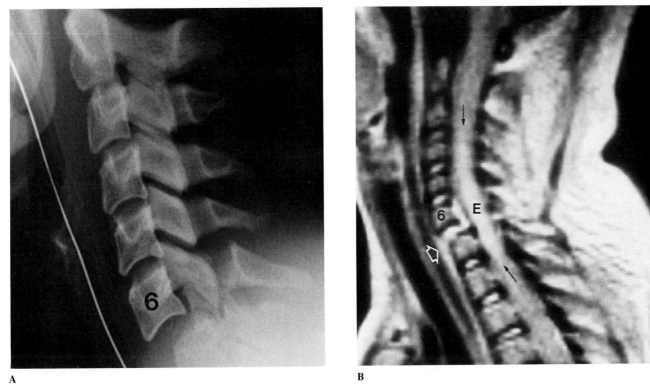

A   B

Figure 3-56 Cord edema after C6-7 dislocation. **(A)** Lateral radiograph shows anterior dislocation of C-6 on C-7. **(B)** Sagittal MRI ($T_R = 2.1$, $T_E = 35$) shows a high-signal area in the spinal cord representing edema (E). Note the cephalad and caudal extent of the edema (thin arrows). Note also the prevertebral, epidural, and intradiskal hemorrhage (open arrow).

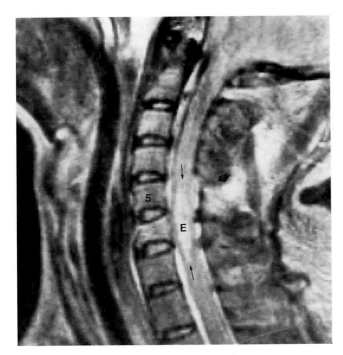

Figure 3-57 Central cord edema (E) in a patient with a C-6 burst fracture. Note the extent of the edema (thin arrows). Note also the posterior soft tissue hemorrhage (wide arrow).

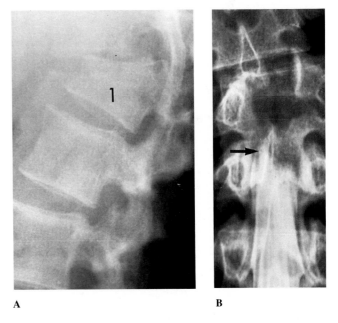

A   B

Figure 3-58 Distraction-type fracture–dislocation of T-12 on L-1. **(A)** Lateral radiograph shows compression of L-1 with dislocation of T-12 over L-1. **(B)** Metrizamide myelogram shows complete obstruction to flow contrast at the L1-2 level (arrow). MRI has nearly completely eliminated the need to perform myelography in vertebral trauma.

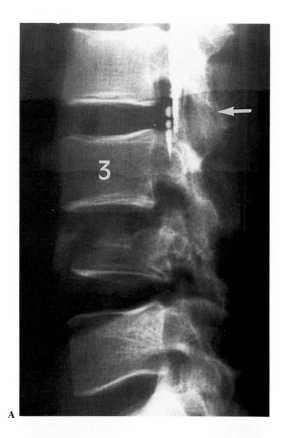

A

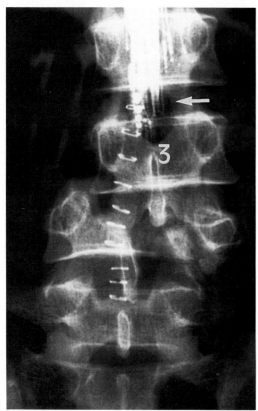

B

Figure 3-59 Pantopaque myelography. The patient suffered a fracture-dis-location involving L-3 and L-4. The column of contrast stops at the L2-3 disk space (arrow), indicating hemorrhage and debris within the vertebral canal at this level. **(A)** Lateral view. **(B)** Frontal view.

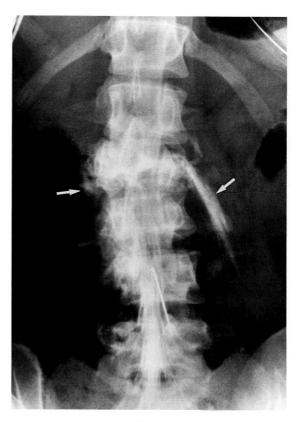

Figure 3-60 Dural tear with extravasation of contrast (arrows) following myelography in a patient with a burst fracture/dislocation of L-2 (same patient as in Fig 3-28).

phy, particularly when combined with CT, is useful for demonstrating extradural lesions, such as herniated intervertebral disks associated with acute skeletal injury (Figs 3-34 and 3-35), the diagnosis of acute traumatic dural tears (Fig 3-60), and the assessment of nerve root avulsions (Fig 3-61).[25,27,28] In addition, this combination is useful for evaluating post-traumatic cystic myelopathy and the development of syringomyelia.[31]

Water-soluble contrast or Pantopaque may be introduced into the subarachnoid space either from the lumbar region or from the atlanto-axial region. Non-ionic water-soluble contrast is the preferred medium, particularly Iohexol or Iopamidol because they have few side effects. The use of water-soluble contrast is generally followed by CT examination (Figs 3-34 and 3-58). If Pantopaque is used, AP and lateral radiographs are obtained after introduction of 1 ml of contrast medium to determine the level of block (Fig 3-59). Air has also been used as a contrast medium by Pay and associates.[27] They found that air myelography was useful for evaluating cervical trauma without bony deformity as well as to delineate thoracic spinal cord in the lateral projection and to demonstrate cord atrophy in the postacute state. The protocol that Pay and associates developed may be used with either air or water-soluble contrast medium if MRI is not available.[27]

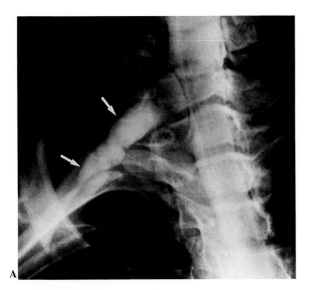
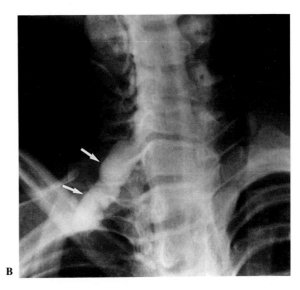

Figure 3-61 Cervical nerve root avulsion C-7. Myelogram spot films show the extravasated contrast along the C-7 nerve root sheath (arrows) (same patient as in Fig 3-36).

REFERENCES

1. Abel MS: The exaggerated supine oblique view of the cervical spine. *Skeletal Radiol* 1982;8:213–219.

2. Acheson MB, Livingston RR, Richardson ML, et al: High-resolution CT scanning in the evaluation of cervical spine fractures: Comparison with plain film examinations. *AJR* 1987;148:1179–1185.

3. Binet EF, Moro JJ, Marangola JP, et al: Cervical spine tomography in trauma. *Spine* 1977;2:163–172.

4. Brant-Zawadzki M, Jeffrey RB, Minagi H, et al: High resolution CT of thoracolumbar fractures. *AJNR* 1982;3:69–74.

5. Brant-Zawadzki M, Miller EM, Federle MP: CT in the evaluation of spine trauma. *AJR* 1981;136:369–375.

6. Chakeres DW, Flickinger F, Bresnahan JC, et al: MR imaging of acute spinal cord trauma. *AJNR* 1987;8:5–10.

7. Daffner RH, Lupetin AR, Dash N, et al: MRI in the detection of malignant infiltration of bone marrow. *AJR* 1986;146:353–358.

8. England AC, Shippel AH, Ray MJ: A simple view for demonstration of fractures of the anterior arch of C-1. *AJR* 1985;144:763–764.

9. Fielding JW, Stillwell WT, Chynn KY, et al: Use of computed tomography for the diagnosis of atlanto-axial rotatory fixation. *J Bone Joint Surg* 1978;60A:1102–1104.

10. Gehweiler JA Jr, Osborne RL Jr, Becker RF: *The Radiology of Vertebral Trauma.* Philadelphia, WB Saunders, 1980.

11. Gellad FE, Levine AM, Joslyn JN, et al: Pure thoracolumbar facet dislocation: Clinical features and CT appearance. *Radiology* 1986;161:505–508.

12. Guerra J Jr, Garfin SR, Resnick D: Vertebral burst fractures: CT analysis of the retropulsed fragment. *Radiology* 1984;153:769–772.

13. Hackney DB, Asato R, Joseph PM, et al: Hemorrhage and edema in acute spinal cord compression: Demonstration by MR imaging. *Radiology* 1986;161:387–390.

14. Handel SF, Lee YY: Computed tomography of spinal fractures. *Radiol Clin North Am* 1981;19:69–89.

15. Harris JH Jr: Radiographic evaluation of spinal trauma. *Orthop Clin North Am* 1986;17:75–86.

16. Harris JH Jr, Edeiken-Monroe B: *The Radiology of Acute Cervical Spine Trauma,* ed 2. Baltimore, Williams & Wilkins, 1987.

17. Kaydoya S, Nakamura T, Kobayashi S, et al: Magnetic resonance imaging of acute spinal cord injury: Report of three cases. *Neuroradiology* 1987;29:252–255.

18. Keene JS, Goletz TH, Lilleas F, et al: Diagnosis of vertebral fractures: A comparison of conventional radiography, conventional tomography and computed axial tomography. *J Bone Joint Surg* 1982;64A:586–594.

19. Kowalski HM, Cohen WA, Cooper P, et al: Pitfalls in the CT diagnosis of atlantoaxial rotary subluxation. *AJNR* 1987;8:697–702.

20. Kulkarni MV, McArdle CB, Kopanicky D, et al: Acute spinal cord injury: MR imaging at 1.5 T. *Radiology* 1987;164:837–843.

21. Manaster BJ, Osborn AG: CT patterns of facet fracture dislocations in the thoracolumbar region. *AJNR* 1986;7:1007–1012.

22. Maravilla KR, Cooper PR, Sklar FH: The influence of thin-section tomography on the treatment of cervical spine injuries. *Radiology* 1978;127:131–139.

23. McArdle CB, Wright JW, Prevost WJ, et al: MR imaging of the acutely injured patient with cervical traction. *Radiology* 1986;159:273–274.

24. Montana MA, Richardson ML, Kilcoyne RF, et al: CT of sacral injury. *Radiology* 1986;161:499–503.

25. Morris RE, Hasso AN, Thompson JR, et al: Traumatic dural tears: CT diagnosis using Metrizamide. *Radiology* 1984;152:443–446.

26. O'Callaghan JP, Ullrich CG, Yuan HA, et al: CT of facet distraction in flexion injuries of the thoracolumbar spine: The ''naked'' facet. *AJNR* 1980;1:97–102.

27. Pay NT, George AE, Benjamin MV, et al: Positive and negative contrast myelography in spinal trauma. *Radiology* 1977;123:103–111.

28. Petras AF, Sobel DF, Mani JR, et al: CT myelography in cervical nerve root avulsion. *J Comput Assist Tomogr* 1985;9(2):275–279.

29. Post MJD, Green BA: The use of computed tomography in spinal trauma. *Radiol Clin North Am* 1983;21:327–375.

30. Post MJD, Green BA, Quencer RM, et al: The value of computed tomography in spinal trauma. *Spine* 1982;7:417–431.

31. Seibert CE, Dreisbach JN, Swanson WB, et al: Progressive post-traumatic cystic myelopathy: Neuroradiologic evaluation. *AJR* 1981;136:1161–1165.

32. Shaffer MA, Doris PE: Limitation of the cross-table lateral view in detecting cervical spine injuries: A retrospective analysis. *Ann Emerg Med* 1981;10:508–513.

33. Steppé R, Bellemans M, Boven F, et al: The value of computed tomography scanning in elusive fractures of the cervical spine. *Skeletal Radiol* 1981;6:175–178.

34. Wojcik WG, Edeiken-Monroe BS, Harris JH Jr: Three-dimensional computed tomography in acute cervical spine trauma: A preliminary report. *Skeletal Radiol* 1987;16:261–269.

35. Yetkin Z, Osborn AG, Giles DS, et al: Uncovertebral and facet joint dislocations in cervical articular pillar fractures: CT evaluation. *AJR* 1985;6:633–637.

Chapter 4

Mechanisms of Injury and Their "Fingerprints"

Vertebral fractures, like fractures in the peripheral skeleton, occur in predictable and reproducible patterns that are related to the kind of force applied to the affected bone. The same force applied to the cervical, thoracic, or lumbar column results in injuries that have a remarkably similar appearance.[7] A review of 1000 injuries to the vertebral column, which the author observed over a 6-year period, suggests that there are essentially four mechanisms of injury: flexion, extension, shearing, and rotation or torque. These injuries may occur as isolated events or in combination with one another. The severity and extent of the damage produced by any one mechanism is dependent on the incident force, the position of the victim at the time of injury, and the victim's velocity. This results in a pattern of recognizable signs that form a spectrum extending from mild soft tissue damage to severe skeletal and ligamentous disruption. The author has termed these patterns the "fingerprints" of the injury.[7] This chapter reviews four basic types of vertebral injury on the basis of their mechanism and the "fingerprints" that result from each.

There are, of course, differences in occurrence of injury based on the relative flexibility and mobility of certain portions of the vertebral column. For example, extension injuries, very common in the cervical region, are relatively rare in the less mobile thoracic and lumbar areas. Lateral flexion injuries in the cervical region tend to produce compression fractures of articular pillars; in the thoracic and lumbar regions, the same forces produce lateral burst injuries of vertebral bodies.

BACKGROUND

The author and his colleagues made the observation that the radiographic changes produced by vertebral injuries had a similar appearance regardless of their location. Two premises were considered: (1) vertebral injuries occur in a predictable pattern that is dependent on mechanism, and (2) vertebral injuries due to a particular mechanism produce the same radiographic changes regardless of location. Just as a criminal leaves fingerprints that link him or her to the crime, the patterns of injury represent the fingerprints that define the full extent of injury. These observations were based on a retrospective and prospective study of 1000 vertebral injuries seen between 1981 and 1986 at the Trauma Center of Allegheny General Hospital in Pittsburgh, Pennsylvania. Of these injuries, 646 (65%) were cervical, 187 (19%) were thoracic, and 167 (16%) were lumbar. Isolated spinous process or transverse process fractures were not included in the study. The levels of injury are indicated in Table 4-1.

Of the 646 cervical injuries, 511 were due to flexion mechanisms, 124 were due to extension, and 11 were purely rotational injuries (rotary luxation of C-2). Of the 187 thoracic injuries, 175 were due to flexion mechanisms. There were no extension injuries. Twelve cases in the thoracolumbar region were shearing injuries, and there were no rotational injuries. Of the 167 lumbar injuries, 165 were due to flexion and 2 were due to extension. These findings are summarized in Table 4-2.

Table 4-1 Vertebral Injuries by Level

Level	Injuries (Number)
C 1	14
2	118
3	48
4	92
5	155
6	134
7	85
Total	646
T 1	18
2	14
3	14
4	16
5	13
6	12
7	10
8	3
9	4
10	8
11	31
12	44
Total	187
L 1	105
2	52
3	6
4	3
5	1
Total	167
Grand Total	1000

Table 4-2 Mechanism of Injury and Level

Level	Mechanism				
	Flexion	Extension	Shear	Rotation	Total
Cervical	511	124	0	11	646
Upper thoracic	87	0	0	0	87
Lower thoracic	25	0	0	0	25
Thoraco-lumbar	216	2	12	2	232
Lower lumbar	10	0	0	0	10
Total	849	126	12	13	1000

FLEXION INJURIES

Flexion injuries may be subdivided into five categories: simple, burst, distraction, dislocation, and combined.

Simple injuries may be defined as compression of the vertebral endplates with anterior wedging of the vertebral body. This injury spares the posterior arch and the posterior ligaments. These injuries are very rarely associated with neurologic deficit (Fig 4-1).

Burst injuries are those in which the vertebra has been exploded by compressive forces, resulting in comminution of the vertebral body, retropulsion of fragments, and cleavage of the posterior arch.[1,15] Injury involves not only the vertebral body but also the posterior arch and the posterior ligaments. These injuries almost always produce severe neurologic deficit (Figs 4-2 and 4-3).

Eighty-five percent of the injuries resulted from motor vehicle accidents. Fourteen percent resulted from falls, and the remaining injuries were results of miscellaneous causes, the most common of which were diving accidents. Those injuries that resulted from motor vehicle accidents were associated, almost universally, with a "deadly triad" of alcohol, high speed (15 miles per hour or more above the posted speed limit), and, in almost all cases of automobile trauma, the absence of seatbelt use.

All patients were evaluated by means of various imaging techniques including plain radiography, computed tomography (CT), polydirectional tomography (PT), and in many instances magnetic resonance imaging (MRI). As mentioned in Chapter 2, the following anatomic regions were defined to take advantage of the natural clustering of injuries at certain levels: cervical, C1-7; upper thoracic, T1-6; lower thoracic, T7-10; thoracolumbar, T11-L2; and lower lumbar, L3-5. Injuries were then categorized on the basis of mechanism: (1) flexion, (2) extension, (3) shearing, (4) rotation or torque, and (5) combined.[11,14,16,21,25] All categories included injuries in which axial loading was a factor.

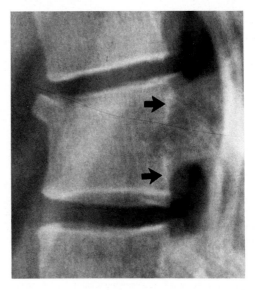

Figure 4-1 Simple compression fracture of L-1. There is anterior wedging of the body of L-1 and a small fragment off the anterosuperior lip of the body of L-1. The posterior vertebral body line (arrows) is intact.

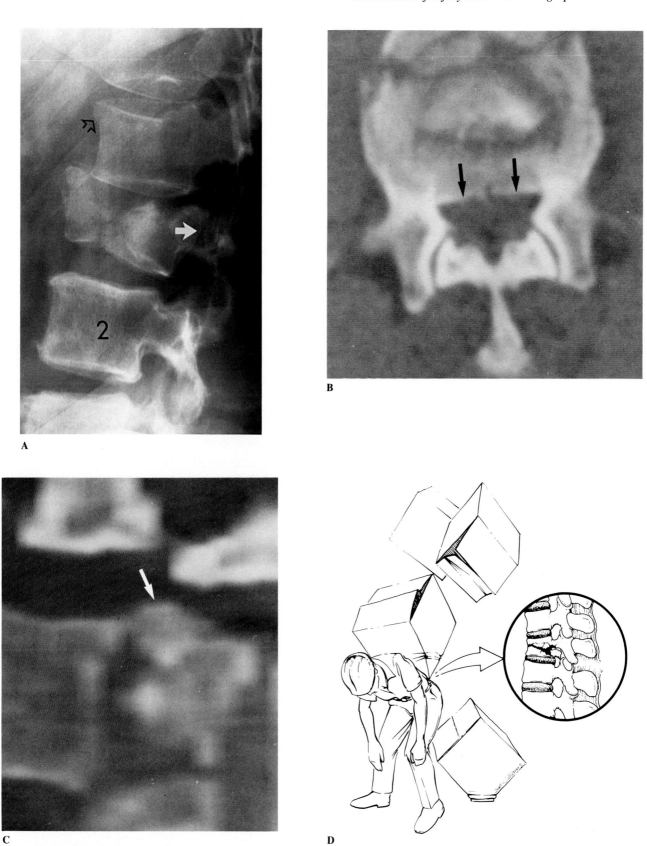

Figure 4-2 Burst fracture of L-1. The patient is paraplegic. Injury resulted from a load of heavy cartons falling on the patient. **(A)** Lateral radiograph shows fragmentation of the body of L-1, narrowing of the T-12 disk space, widening of the L-1 disk space, and retropulsion of a bony fragment posteriorly (solid arrow). In addition, there is a simple compression fracture of the body of T-12 (open arrow). **(B)** CT scan shows severe comminution of the body of L-1 with retropulsion of two bony fragments that have narrowed the vertebral canal (arrows). **(C)** Sagittal reconstruction of the CT scan shows a retropulsed bony fragment within the vertebral canal (arrow). Compare with **(A)**. **(D)** Drawing of the mechanism of injury in this patient.

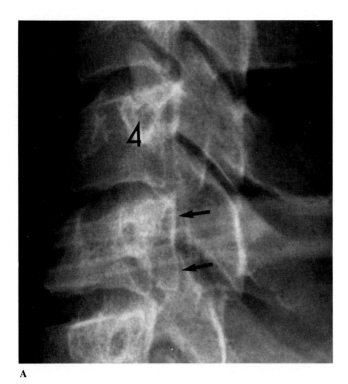

A

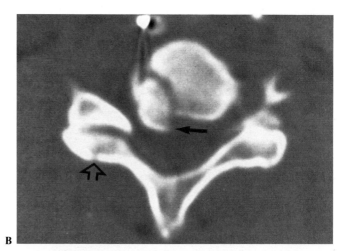

B

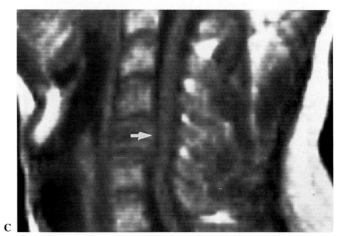

C

Figure 4-3 Cervical burst fracture. The patient is quadriplegic. **(A)** Lateral radiograph shows retropulsed fragment of bone from the body of C-5 (arrows). Note the gaping of the facet joints of C5-6 as a further indicator of a flexion mechanism. **(B)** CT scan through the area shows the large fragment of the body of C-5 that has been retropulsed into the vertebral canal (thin arrow). In addition, there is a fracture of the articular pillar on the right (open arrow). **(C)** MRI ($T_R = 0.3$, $T_E = 35$) shows the canal compromise with spinal cord encroachment (arrow).

Distraction injuries are those that result in widening of the interspinous and interfacet distance without frank dislocation. There may be associated fractures due to avulsion of bony elements. These injuries also tend to produce neurologic deficit in a high percentage of cases (Fig 4-4).

Dislocation injuries are those in which there is a loss of bony continuity at articular surfaces. In the cervical region, facet lock is a common manifestation of this injury. These injuries also tend to result in a high incidence of neurologic deficit (Figs 4-5 and 4-6).

Combined injuries are those with features of more than one of the above categories (Fig 4-7).

Flexion injuries are the most common of all vertebral injuries. They may occur as an isolated event or, more commonly, in combination with axial loading. Not surprisingly, motor vehicle accidents account for most flexion injuries. In the most typical scenario, an unrestrained occupant of a motor vehicle strikes the vertex of the head on a solid object. In the case of the driver or the front seat passenger this object is the windshield (Fig 4-8). In the case of a rear seat passenger, the object is usually the roof. Both these mechanisms are considered "ejection" injuries. In another mechanism involving occu-

pants of a motor vehicle, particularly one that rolls over, the victim strikes the head and hyperflexes the neck on any other solid object within the vehicle. In many of these individuals a devastating vertebral injury could easily have been avoided by the use of seatbelts.

Cervical injuries produced by this mechanism are usually clustered between C-5 and C-7. Flexion injuries to the thoracolumbar region have also been found in drivers of motor vehicles who struck the steering column, which serves as a fulcrum for flexion.

Once an individual is thrown from a motor vehicle, flexion injuries may occur at any level within the vertebral column when the victim strikes a solid object and the body flexes. This particular mechanism accounts for many of the two-level injuries (cervical-thoracic, cervical-lumbar, thoracic-lumbar) that have been observed by a number of investigators.[3,14]

Occupants of motor vehicles who wear lap-type seatbelts may suffer a unique type of distraction fracture. Although originally described by Smith and Chance, these are generically referred to as Chance fractures (Fig 4-9). In these injuries, the lap belt becomes the fulcrum of flexion at the anterior abdominal wall.[4,24] The vertebra is literally ripped in two

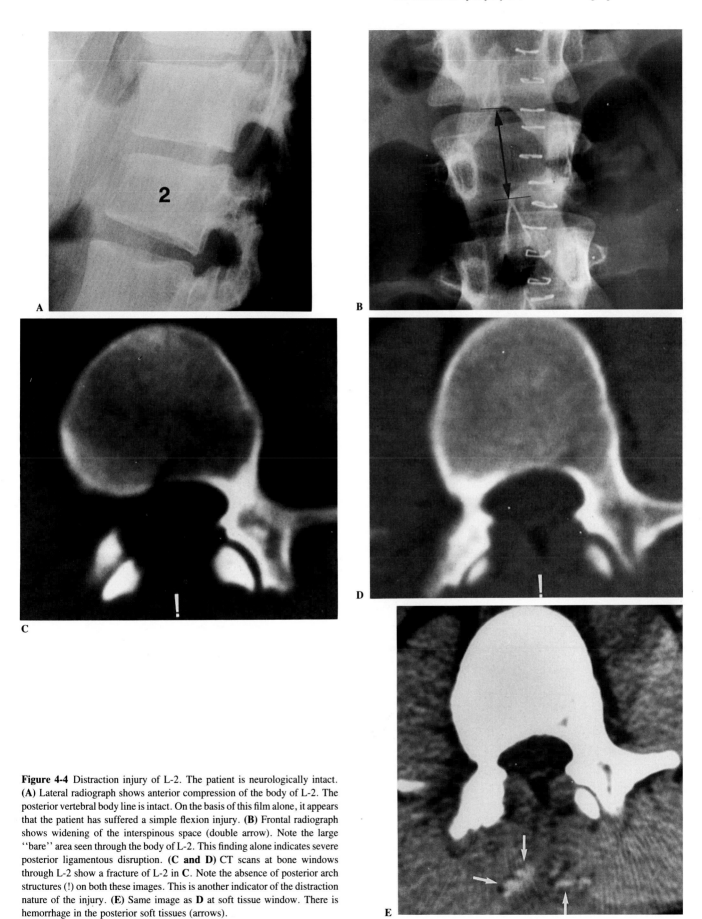

Figure 4-4 Distraction injury of L-2. The patient is neurologically intact. **(A)** Lateral radiograph shows anterior compression of the body of L-2. The posterior vertebral body line is intact. On the basis of this film alone, it appears that the patient has suffered a simple flexion injury. **(B)** Frontal radiograph shows widening of the interspinous space (double arrow). Note the large "bare" area seen through the body of L-2. This finding alone indicates severe posterior ligamentous disruption. **(C and D)** CT scans at bone windows through L-2 show a fracture of L-2 in **C**. Note the absence of posterior arch structures (!) on both these images. This is another indicator of the distraction nature of the injury. **(E)** Same image as **D** at soft tissue window. There is hemorrhage in the posterior soft tissues (arrows).

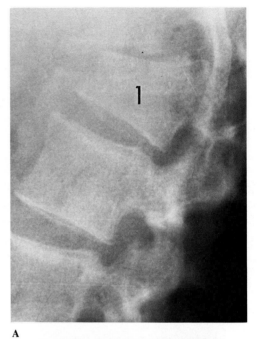

A

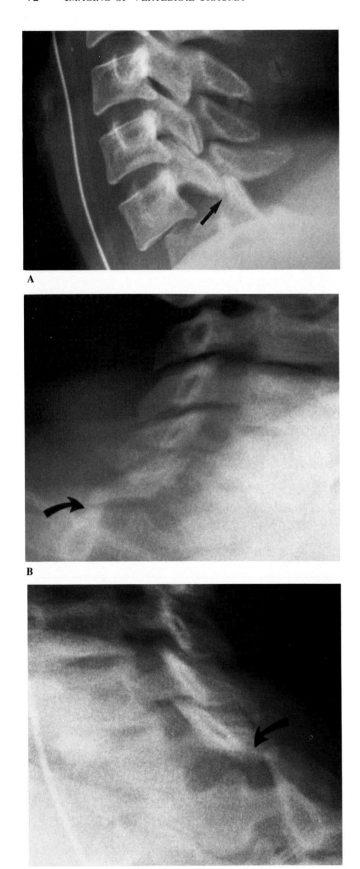

A

B

C

Figure 4-5 Cervical dislocation with bilateral locked facets of C-6 on C-7. The arrows show the locking. (A) Lateral radiograph. (B and C) Trauma oblique views.

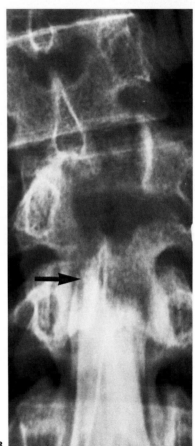

B

Figure 4-6 Thoracolumbar dislocation of T-12 on L-1 with fracture of L-1. The patient is paraplegic. (A) Lateral radiograph shows anterior dislocation of T-12 on L-1. There is anterior compression of L-1. The posterior vertebral body line of L-1 is indistinct superiorly, suggesting retropulsion of a bone fragment. (B) Metrizamide myelogram shows complete obstruction to the flow of contrast material at the L1-2 region (arrow) in addition to the dislocation of T-12 on L-1 and the fracture through the pedicle of L-1 on the left.

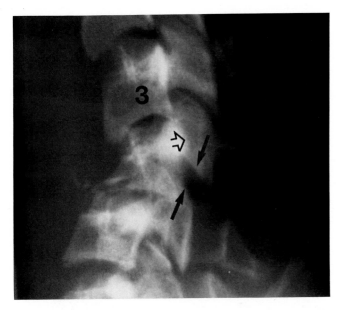

Figure 4-7 Combined cervical flexion injury as a result of an automobile accident. There is total disruption of the body of C-4. A small fragment of bone has been retropulsed into the vertebral canal (open arrow). Note the widening of the facet joints (solid arrows). All these findings indicate a combination of burst and distraction. The overall malalignment is the result of dislocation.

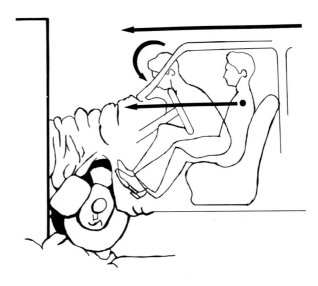

Figure 4-8 Flexion mechanism in an unrestrained motor vehicle driver. On impact, the victim pitches forward. The chest is impaled on the steering column. The knees strike the dashboard. This mechanism is sufficient to produce flexion injuries in the lumbar vertebrae. In addition, if the head pitches forward, flexion injury may result as contact is made with the windshield.

through a horizontal plane (Fig 4-10). The thoracolumbar region is most commonly involved. These injuries generally result in severe neurologic deficit.

A similar injury is produced when an individual traveling at a high rate of speed (either from a fall or while skiing) strikes a solid object with the upper abdomen and the trunk forcibly flexes over that fulcrum (Fig 4-11).

Motorcyclists suffer a characteristic fracture in the upper thoracic region when they are ejected over the handlebars and contact a solid object. In most instances, the area of contact is in the upper thorax between the scapulae. These injuries characteristically involve dislocations between T-2 and T-6 (Figs 4-12 and 4-13).

Individuals who dive into shallow water suffer a devastating injury of the lower cervical region, usually at the C5-7 level (Figs 4-14 and 4-15). In this case, the weight of the body provides the axial loading force that causes the damage.[14]

Another form of flexion mechanism occurs in individuals who jump or fall from a height and land on their feet.[12] In addition to the calcaneal fractures, the resultant forward flexion with the axial load of the upper torso generally produces burst fractures in the thoracolumbar region. Individuals with a history of a fall or with known bilateral calcaneal fractures should have radiographs of the thoracolumbar region.

On the basis of the radiographic features encountered, the author and his colleagues were able to categorize the 849 flexion injuries as follows: simple, 130; burst, 185; distraction, 37; dislocation, 233; and combined, 264.[7] Simple inju-

ries were most common in the cervical and upper thoracic regions. Burst fractures were most common in the thoracolumbar region. Surprisingly, however, there were a significant number of burst injuries in the lower cervical region (C5-7). Pure distraction injuries were unusual and occurred in the cervical and thoracolumbar areas only. Dislocation was most common in the cervical region. All cases of unilateral or bilateral facet lock were included in this group. Table 4-3 summarizes these data and lists the type of injury by location.

Flexion injuries characteristically involve the vertebral bodies, the apophyseal (facet) joints, and the posterior ligaments. Fractures of the bony posterior elements are secondary to injuries of these structures. An exception is the "clay shoveler" fracture of the spinous process of the lower cervical column, which occurs as an isolated injury (Fig 4-16).

The fingerprints of flexion injuries include compression (Fig 4-17), fragmentation (Fig 4-18) and burst fracture of vertebral bodies (Figs 4-19 and 4-20), "teardrop" fragments of the inferior lips of vertebral bodies (Fig 4-21), widening of the interspinous or interlaminar spaces (Figs 4-19 and 4-22), anterolisthesis (Fig 4-23), disruption of the posterior vertebral body line (Figs 4-19 and 4-20), jumped or locked facets (Figs 4-24 and 4-25), and narrowing of the intervertebral disk spaces, usually above and below the level of involvement (Figs 4-17 and 4-22).[7,14] Once again, it is important to emphasize that these findings may be seen at any level of the vertebral column. Note the similarity among findings in Figs 4-19 and 4-20.

(text continues on p. 80)

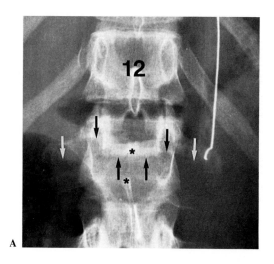

A

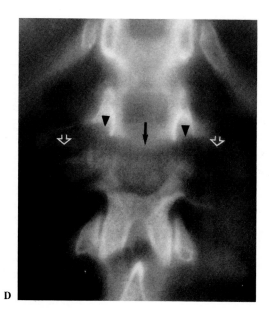

D

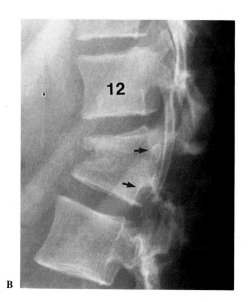

B

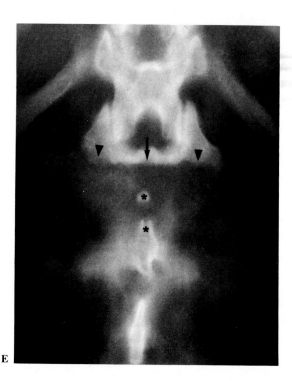

E

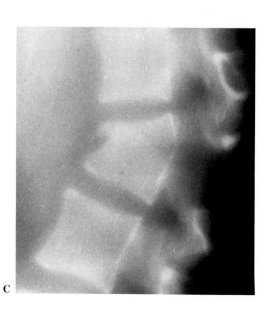

C

Figure 4-9 Horizontal vertebral injury in a rear seat passenger wearing a lap-type seatbelt (Chance fracture). **(A)** Frontal radiograph shows overall increase in the height of L-1. The fracture lines extending through the transverse processes, pedicles, and laminae are easily identifiable (arrows). The spinous process is cleft in two (*). **(B)** Lateral radiograph shows horizontal cleavage through L-1 with posterior bowing and gaping of the vertebral body (arrows). **(C)** Lateral tomogram shows findings similar to those in **B** in better detail. **(D and E)** Frontal tomograms show the horizontal nature of the fracture extending through the transverse processes (open arrows), pedicles (arrowheads), and laminae (solid arrow). In D, note the fracture in the spinous process (*).

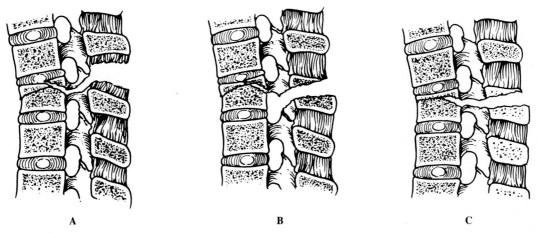

Figure 4-10 Three types of flexion injuries due to the use of lap-type seatbelts. **(A)** Smith fracture. **(B)** Chance fracture. **(C)** Pure horizontal fracture. *Source:* Reprinted from ''Injuries of Thoracolumbar Vertebral Column'' by RH Daffner, in *Radiology in Emergency Medicine* by MK Dalinka and JJ Kaye (Eds) with permission of Churchill Livingstone Inc., © 1984.

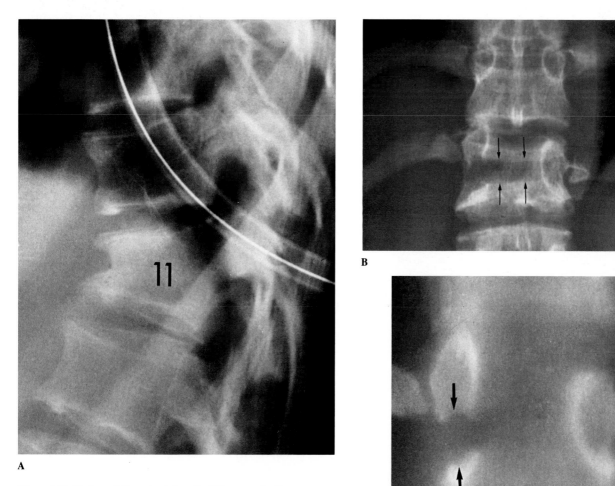

Figure 4-11 Horizontal distraction injury (Smith) as a result of lap-type seatbelt use in a rear seat passenger. **(A)** Lateral radiograph shows anterior compression of T-11 and posterior distraction. **(B)** Frontal radiograph shows the cleft in T-11. The horizontal fracture is easily seen (arrows). The fracture involves the pedicle on the right side. Note the increased distance between the 11th and 12th ribs, particularly on the right. **(C)** Frontal tomogram through the pedicle region shows the fractures on the right (arrows). Note the elevation of the superior aspect of the pedicle on the right side.

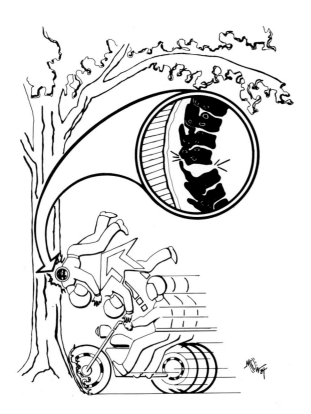

Figure 4-12 Mechanism of flexion injury in motorcyclists. On impact with a solid object, the rider is thrown over the handlebars. Forward flexion occurs in the high thoracic region. *Source:* Reprinted with permission from "Thoracic Fractures and Dislocations in Motorcyclists" by RH Daffner et al in *Skeletal Radiology* (1987;16:280–284), Copyright © 1987, Springer-Verlag.

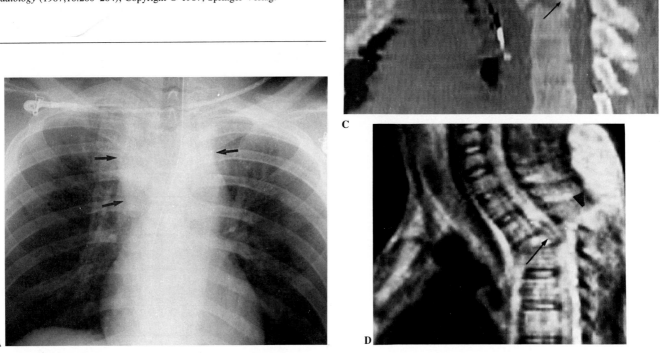

Figure 4-13 High thoracic fracture-dislocation in a motorcyclist. The patient is paraplegic. **(A)** Chest radiograph shows widening of the mediastinum posteriorly (arrows). **(B)** CT scan through the T-3 region shows bony fragments within the vertebral canal. There is posterior fragmentation as well. Note the bilateral pleural effusion and mediastinal widening. **(C)** Sagittal reconstruction shows a large bony fragment from T-3 within the vertebral canal (arrow). There is posterior dislocation. **(D)** MRI ($T_R = 0.3$, $T_E = 35$) shows similar findings with a large bony fragment virtually transecting the spinal cord at T-3 (arrow). Note the posterior hemorrhage, which manifests as high signal (arrowhead). *Source:* Reprinted with permission from "Thoracic Fractures and Dislocations in Motorcyclists" by RH Daffner et al in *Skeletal Radiology* (1987;16:280–284), Copyright © 1987, Springer-Verlag.

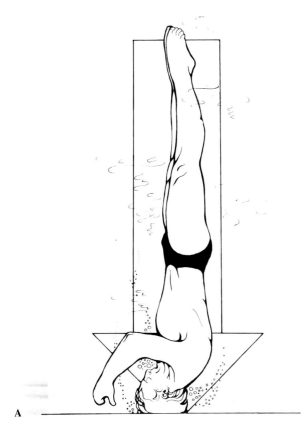

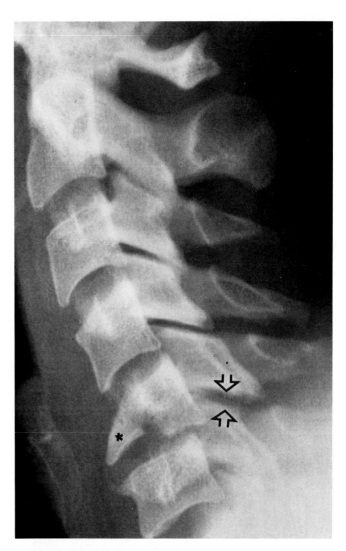

Figure 4-15 "Teardrop" fracture of C-5 from a diving accident. There is posterior dislocation of C-5 on C-6. Note the "teardrop" fragment (*). As further evidence of flexion injury, there is widening of the facet joints of C5-6 (open arrows). There is also widening of the interspinous space.

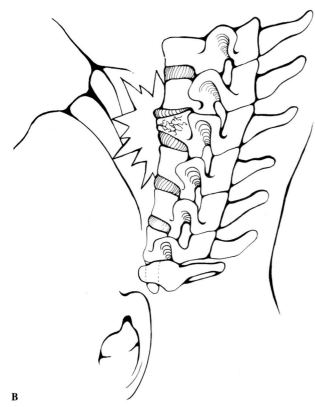

Figure 4-14 Mechanism of flexion injury in diving accidents. The diver's head strikes the bottom with resultant forced flexion and increase in axial load. This mechanism characteristically produces a "teardrop" fracture, usually at C-5.

Table 4-3 Flexion Injuries

| Level | Injury | | | | | |
	Simple	Burst	Distraction	Dislocation	Combined	Total
Cervical	43	58	19	174	215	509
Upper thoracic	47	18	0	15	6	86
Lower thoracic	11	5	0	3	3	22
Thoraco-lumbar	18	104	18	41	40	221
Lower lumbar	11	0	0	0	0	11
Total	130	185	37	233	264	849

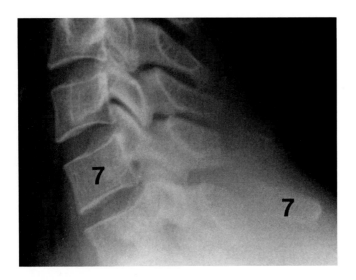

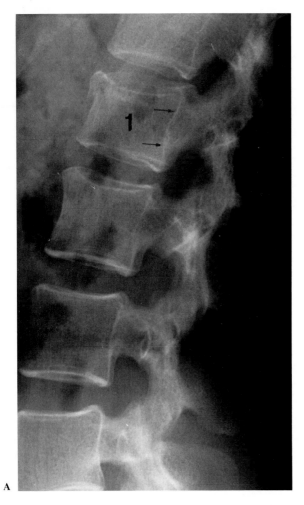

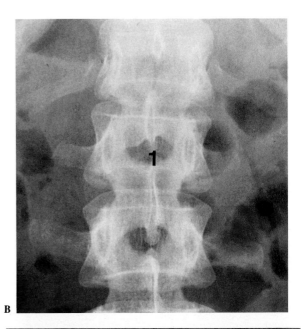

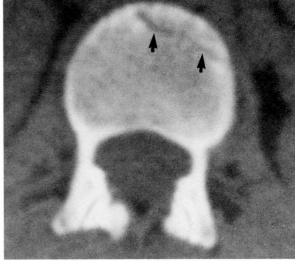

Figure 4-16 ''Clay-shoveler'' fractures of C-7 and T-1. The fractured spinous process of C-7 has been displaced downward due to muscular pull. Lateral tomograms showed a similar fracture of T-1.

Figure 4-17 Simple compression fracture of L-1. The patient is neurologically intact. **(A)** Lateral radiograph shows compression of the anterosuperior lip of L-1. The posterior vertebral body line (arrows) is intact. **(B)** Frontal radiograph shows compression of the body of L-1. The interspinous distance is normal. **(C)** CT scan shows a fracture of the anterosuperior lip of L-1 (arrows). The posterior vertebral body line is intact.

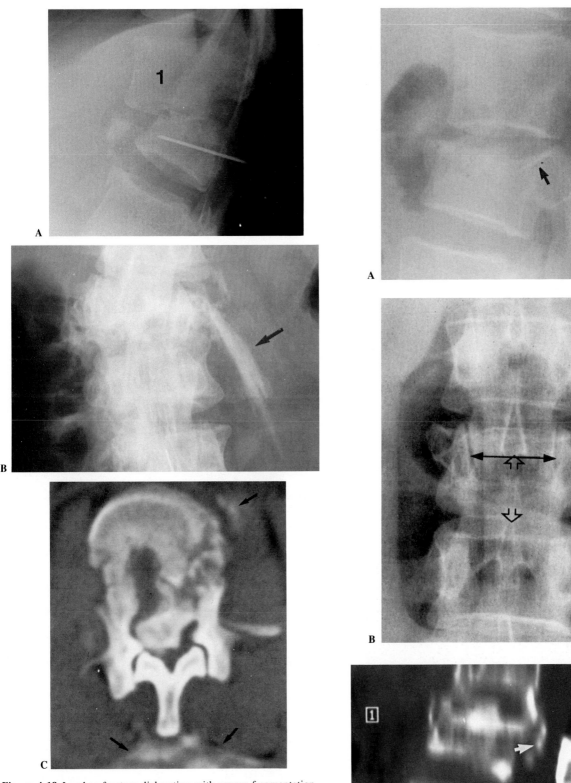

Figure 4-18 Lumbar fracture-dislocation with severe fragmentation. **(A)** Lateral radiograph shows dislocation of L-1 on L-2. There is marked fragmentation of the body of L-2. There is also a simple fracture of the anterosuperior aspect of the body of L-3. **(B)** Frontal radiograph after Metrizamide myelography shows extravasation of contrast material at L-2 (arrow). Note the total disruption in alignment as a result of the fracture of L-2. **(C)** CT scan shows fragmentation of the body of L-2 with a large central fragment displaced into the vertebral canal. Extravasated contrast material from the myelogram is present anteriorly as well as posteriorly (arrows).

Figure 4-19 Burst fracture of L-3. **(A)** Lateral radiograph shows compression of the body of L-3 anteriorly. There has been posterior displacement of a bony fragment (arrow). **(B)** Frontal radiograph shows widening of the interspinous space (open arrow) as well as widening of the interpedicular distance (double arrow). **(C)** CT scan sagittal reconstruction shows a large bony fragment encroaching on the vertebral canal (arrow).

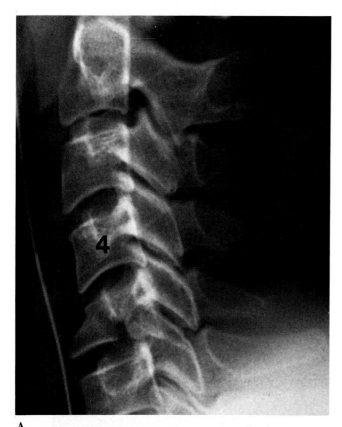

A

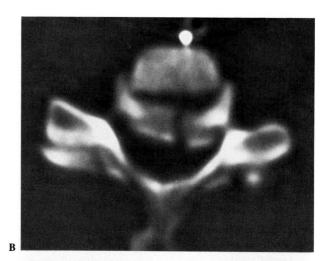

B

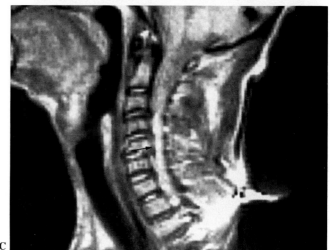

C

Figure 4-20 Cervical burst fracture due to a diving accident. **(A)** Lateral radiograph shows disruption of the body of C-5 with posterior displacement of the posterior half of the body of C-5. There is slight widening of the facet joints of C5-6. **(B)** CT scan shows marked canal compromise at C-5 by two large bony fragments. **(C)** MRI ($T_R = 0.1$, $T_E = 35$) shows the canal compromise (arrow). The area of high signal indicates hemorrhage within the spinal cord.

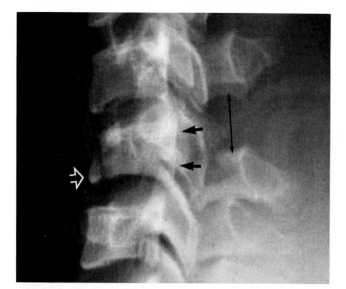

Figure 4-21 Cervical combined flexion injury due to a diving accident. There is a small "teardrop" fragment anteroinferiorly (open arrow). A bony fragment has been displaced posteriorly to encroach on the vertebral canal (solid arrows). In addition, there is widening of the interlaminar space (double arrow).

EXTENSION INJURIES

Extension injuries may be divided into three categories: simple, distraction, and dislocation.[2,11,14,16,21–23,25]

Simple injuries are defined as avulsion of the anterosuperior portion of the vertebral body. They produce minimal radiographic findings and often result in severe neurologic deficit (Figs 4-26 and 4-27).

Distraction injuries are those that result in widening of the intervertebral disk space with or without an avulsion fracture of the vertebral body below.[2] The "hangman" fracture of C-2 with separation of the fracture fragments is also an example of a distraction injury (Figs 4-28 to 4-30).[22,23] In the former case, there is usually severe neurologic deficit; in the latter, there is generally no neurologic deficit.

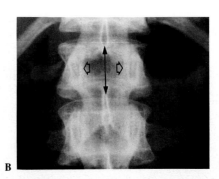

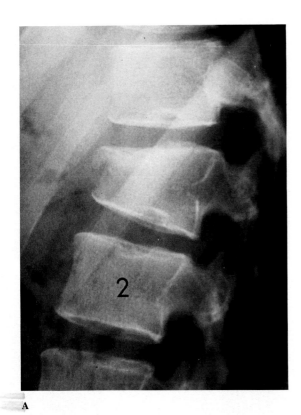

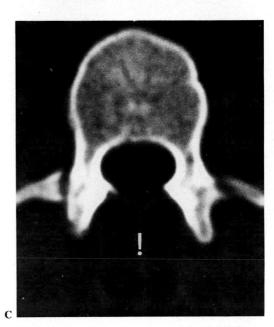

Figure 4-22 Wide interspinous space. **(A)** Lateral radiograph shows an apparent simple compression fracture of L-1. **(B)** Frontal radiograph shows widening of the interspinous space (double arrow). In addition, the facets of L-1 are "naked" (open arrows). These two findings indicate posterior distraction of the vertebra. **(C)** CT scan through L-1 shows absence of articulating element of T-12. Note the large bare area posteriorly (!).

Dislocation is loss of bony continuity at the articular surfaces. These injuries almost always produce severe neurologic deficit.

Extension injuries are extremely common in the cervical column and rare in the thoracic and lumbar regions. Of 126 extension injuries encountered in the author's study, 124 occurred in the cervical region. Most of these were at C-2, where there was a bilateral traumatic spondylolysis ("hangman" fracture). The remaining two were in the thoracolumbar region. One of these occurred in a patient with ankylosing spondylitis who injured his back in a fall; the other occurred in an individual who fell backward, extending himself across a metal bar. Table 4-4 summarizes these data.

Extension injuries occur in various circumstances. In the cervical region, two of the most commonly encountered mechanisms are automobile accidents and falls. In an automobile

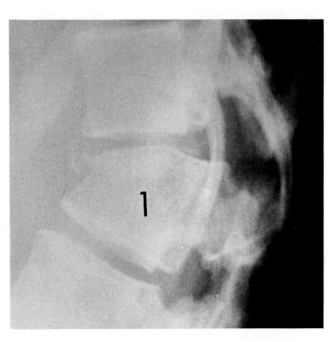

Figure 4-23 Anterolisthesis of T-12 on L-1 due to flexion injury.

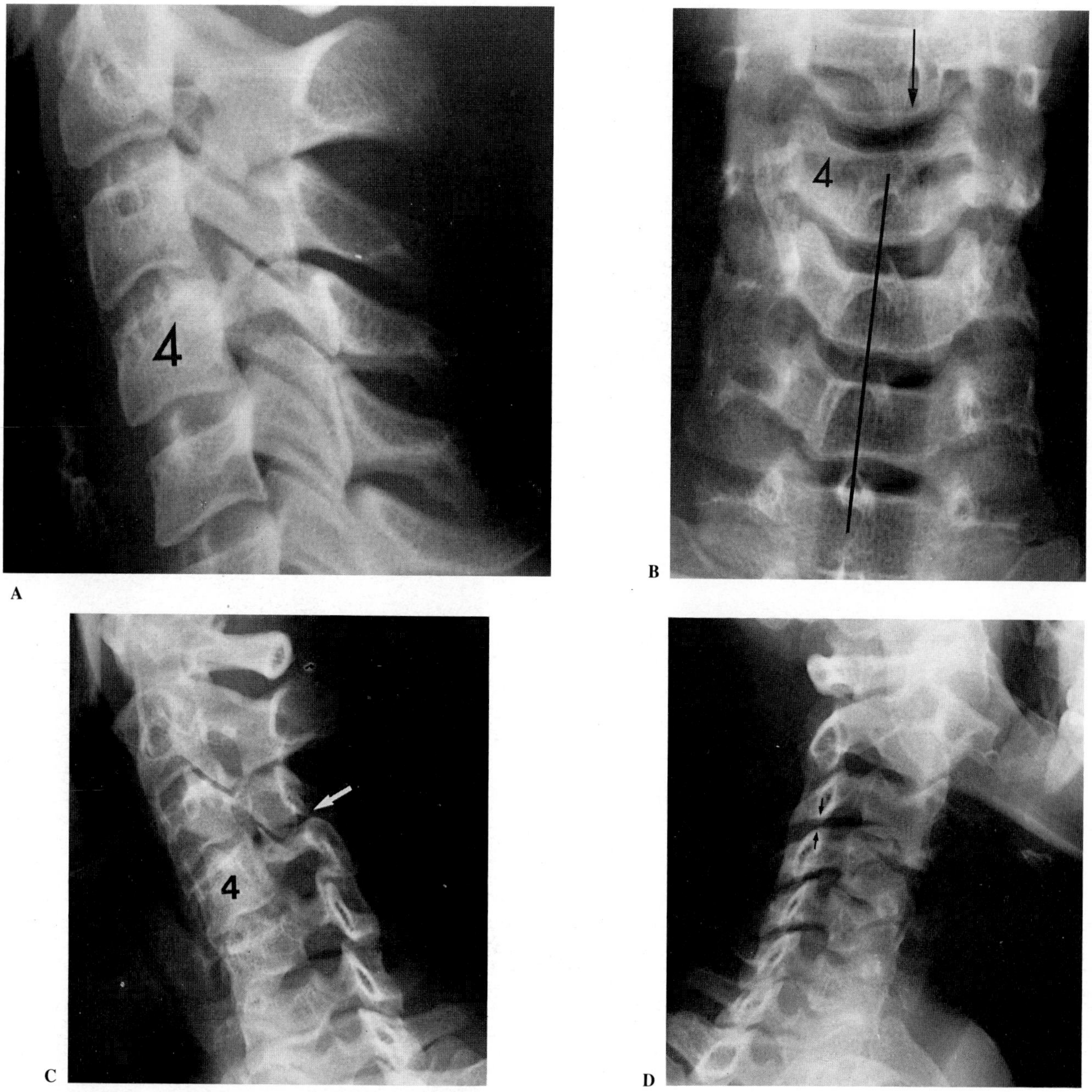

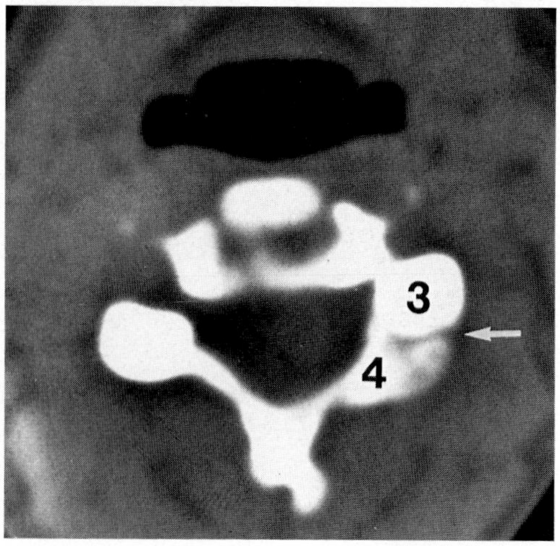

Figure 4-24 Unilateral facet lock at the C3-4 disk space. (**A**) Lateral radiograph shows duplication of facet shadows at C-3 and C-4. The overall alignment of the vertebral bodies appears to be normal. (**B**) Frontal radiograph shows malalignment of the spinous processes at C-3 and C-4. The spinous process of C-3 is rotated to the left (arrow). The spinous processes of C-4 through C-7 align (straight line). (**C**) Left oblique radiograph shows the point of locking of the facets of C-3 and C-4 (arrow). (**D**) Right oblique radiograph shows normal alignment on the right side. There is, however, widening of the facet joint of C3-4 on the right (arrows) as a result of the locking on the left. (**E**) CT scan shows the point of locking on the left (arrow).

accident, the unrestrained driver's neck may be hyperextended as the chest strikes the steering wheel, producing a traumatic spondylolysis of the posterior arch of C-2 ("hangman" fracture) (Fig 4-29).[14,16,22,23] Fractures of the dens with posterior dislocation may also occur with extension (anterior fracture-dislocation of the dens usually occurs with a flexion mechanism). It is unusual for either of these extension injuries to have any associated neurologic findings. These injuries may produce nothing more clinically than upper neck stiffness, dysphagia, or torticollis. The patients may seek clinical evaluation days or weeks after injury (Figs 4-28 and 4-30).

A second extension-type injury in the cervical region occurs at a lower level. Anatomically, these may range from simple hyperextension sprains, in which the anterior ligaments are disrupted along with disk-bond injury (Fig 4-31),[5,14,20] to severe fracture-dislocation (Fig 4-32). In either case, the patient may have severe neurologic compromise. This is particularly true in elderly individuals in whom osteophytes project posteriorly into the vertebral canal. In these individuals, relatively mild extension trauma may result in severe neurologic compromise. The typical clinical findings involve an elderly patient with quadriplegia in whom the only significant radiologic finding is cervical spondylosis.

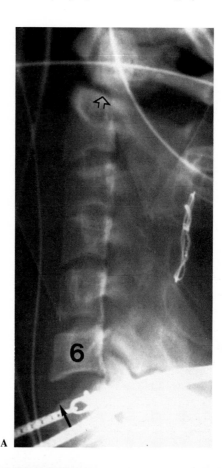

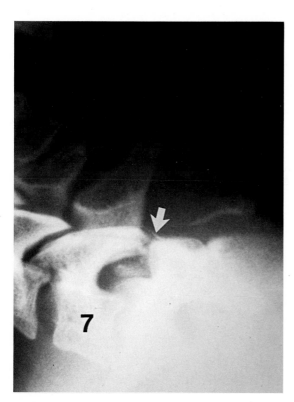

Figure 4-25 Bilateral jumped locked facets at the C7-T1 disk space. The patient is neurologically intact. The point of locking is indicated by the arrow. An avulsed portion of the spinous process of C-7 lies just to the right of the arrow.

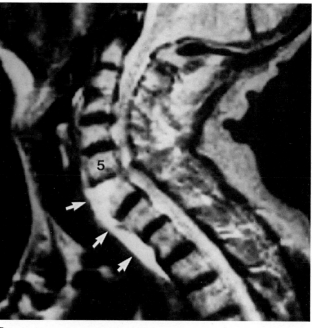

Figure 4-26 Extension injuries. **(A)** Lateral radiograph shows a fracture of the base of the dens with retrolisthesis (open arrow). In addition, there is widening of the anterior vertebral disk space of C-6. Note the vacuum phenomenon just above the body of C-7 (solid arrow). This vacuum sign is further evidence of an extension mechanism. **(B)** MRI (T_R = 2.1, T_E = 90) in another patient with a similar injury at C5-6. There is widening of the C-5 disk space. The area of high signal at C-5 and below (arrows) represents hemorrhage in the prevertebral space. This patient is quadriplegic.

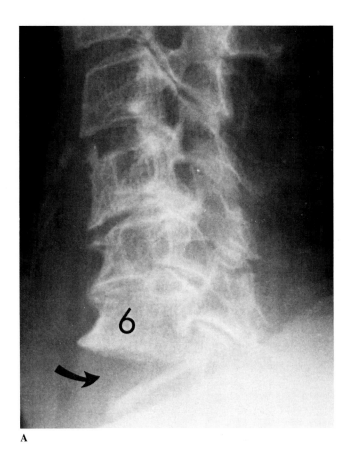

A

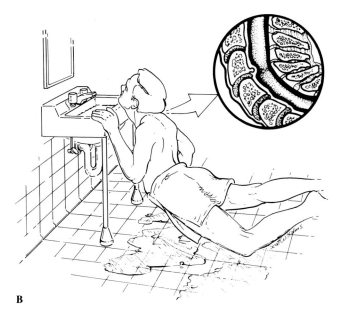

B

Figure 4-27 Distraction-type extension injury at C6-7 in an elderly patient. **(A)** Note the widening of the C-6 disk space (arrow). The patient is quadriplegic. **(B)** Mechanism of this extension injury. Forced extension of the cervical vertebral column produces severe cord compromise as a result of compression of the spinal cord by osteophytes. This is a common mechanism of injury in a severely neurologically compromised elderly patient in whom the only radiographic finding is evidence of degenerative joint disease.

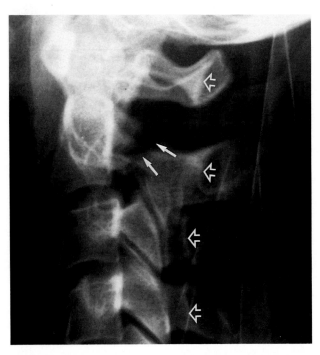

Figure 4-28 "Hangman" fracture of C-2 (solid arrows). Note the disruption of the spinolaminar line resulting from anterolisthesis of the body of C-2 and C-1 (open arrows).

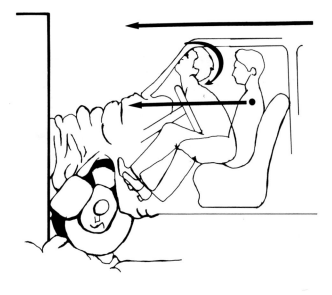

Figure 4-29 Mechanism of "hangman" injury in an automobile accident. The unrestrained driver pitches forward, impaling the thorax on the steering wheel. If the face strikes the windshield before the vertex of the head, the head is forced backward in hyperextension. This produces the cervical injury.

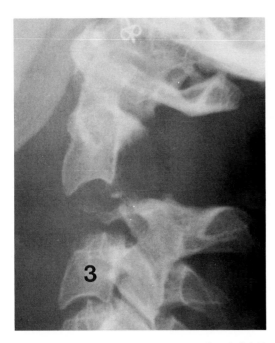

Figure 4-30 "Hangman" fracture as it would appear after a judicial hanging. In addition to the fracture of the posterior arch of C-2, there is wide distraction of C-2 from C-3 with subsequent tearing of the spinal cord.

Table 4-4 Extension Injuries

Level	Injury			Total
	Simple	Distraction	Dislocation	
Cervical	65	7	52	124
Thoracic	0	0	0	0
Lumbar	0	2	0	2
Total	65	9	52	126

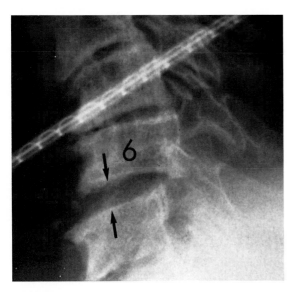

Figure 4-31 Extension sprain. In this elderly individual, there is widening of the C-6 disk space (arrows) and retrolisthesis of the vertebral column above C-6. This resulted in quadriplegia.

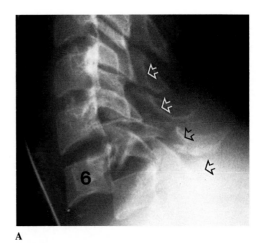

A

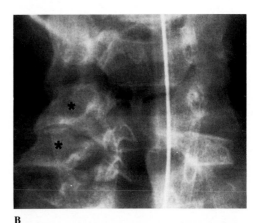

B

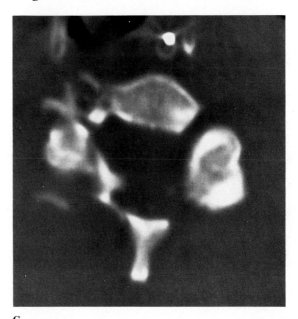

C

Figure 4-32 Hyperextension fracture-dislocation (Gehweiler type V). **(A)** Lateral radiograph shows anterolisthesis of all the vertebrae from C-6 and above over C-7. There is apparent locking of the facets of C-6 on C-7. Note, however, that the spinolaminar line is essentially unbroken (arrows). This serves to differentiate this injury from a flexion-type injury. **(B)** Frontal radiograph shows malalignment of the pillars of C-5 and C-6 (*), indicating that they are free floating. **(C)** CT scan shows widening of the vertebral canal and fragmentation of the entire vertebra.

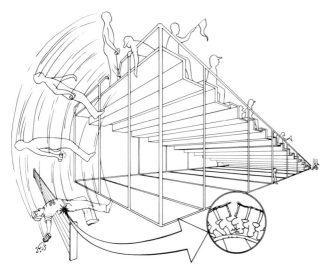

Figure 4-33 Mechanism of extension injury of the thoracolumbar vertebral column. Most of these injuries occur when the individual falls and lands across a fixed object, as in this drawing. A similar injury may occur in individuals who are thrown from a motorcycle or a horse and strike a solid object.

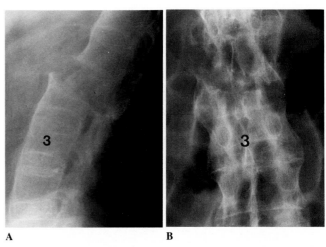

Figure 4-35 Extension injury of L-2 in a patient with ankylosing spondylitis. **(A)** Lateral radiograph shows disruption of L-2 and retrolisthesis of the vertebrae above L-2. **(B)** Frontal radiograph shows the transection of L-2 as a result of the fracture. Malalignment is present. Note the changes of ankylosing spondylitis on both these radiographs.

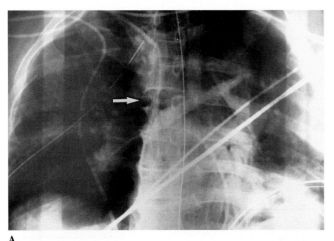

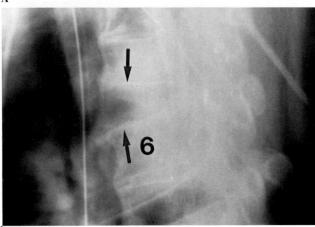

Figure 4-34 Extension injury of T5-6 in a patient with diffuse idiopathic skeletal hyperostosis (DISH) who fell a distance of 30 feet from a bridge. **(A)** Frontal radiograph shows widening of the T5-6 disk space (arrow). There are numerous pieces of life-support equipment present. **(B)** Lateral radiograph shows gaping of the T5-6 interspace (arrows). Note the changes of DISH on both films.

Extension injuries are highly unusual in the thoracic and lumbar regions. They may occur, however, in several circumstances. In one, an individual falls and hyperextends over a solid object (Fig 4-33). In another, the individual is struck from behind by a large object with resultant hyperextension (Fig 4-34). In extremely rare circumstances, an individual with ankylosing spondylitis may suffer an extension injury through the fused vertebrae with relatively minor trauma (Figs 4-35 and 4-36).[26]

The fingerprints of an extension injury include widening of the disk space below the level of injury (Fig 4-31) and triangular avulsion fractures of the anterosuperior lip of vertebral bodies (Figs 4-26 and 4-31), retrolisthesis (Fig 4-31), neural arch fractures (Fig 4-30), and, in the less common extension fracture-dislocation involving the articular pillars and vertebral arches (Gehweiler type IV and V fractures), anterolisthesis with normal interspinous or interlaminar spaces and normal spinolaminar lines (Fig 4-32).[7]

SHEARING INJURIES

Shearing injuries are the result of horizontally directed forces in which axial loading is not a factor. They may occur in combination with flexion or extension injuries. In most instances, the lower portion of the body is fixed; in the unfixed portion, the vertebral column absorbs the horizontal force and moves with it (Figs 4-37 and 4-38).[7,14] The fingerprints of shearing injuries are discussed below. These injuries are generally severely disruptive, and almost all are associated with significant neurologic compromise.

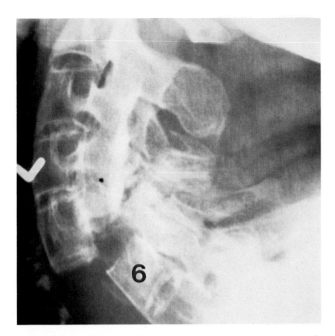

Figure 4-36 Ankylosing spondylitis in a patient who suffered a fracture-dislocation of C5-6 after striking his chin on a coffee table. As with Fig 4-32, the spinolaminar line remains relatively intact.

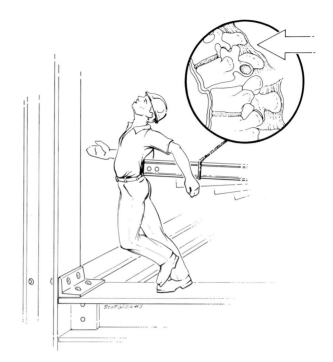

Figure 4-37 Mechanism of shearing injury.

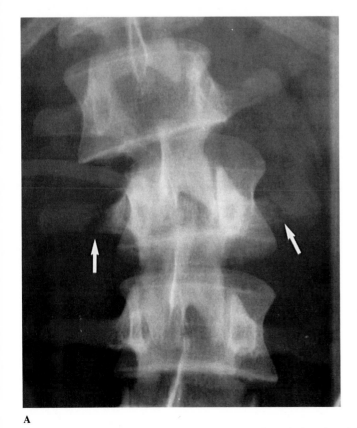

A

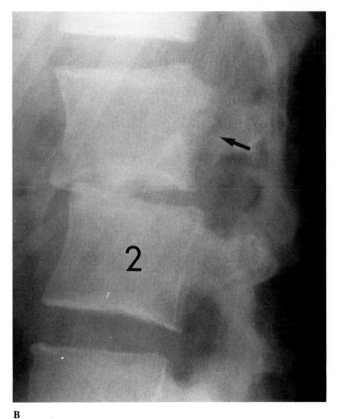

B

Figure 4-38 Pure shearing injury of L1-2. (**A**) Frontal radiograph shows lateral displacement of the vertebrae above L-2 to the right. Note the transverse process fractures of L-2 (arrows). (**B**) Lateral radiograph shows disruption of the L1-2 disk space. There is anteriolisthesis of L-1 on L-2. A pedicle fracture (subsequently shown to be bilateral) is present (arrow).

ROTATIONAL (TORQUE) INJURIES

Rotational injuries result from a rotary or torsion force applied about the long axis of the vertebral column. They are commonly associated with a flexion mechanism as a result of vertebral loading or compression in the thoracolumbar region from above. The usual mechanism is that of a heavy blow in the shoulder region that compresses the vertebral column while deflecting the torso laterally. This results in disruption of the posterior ligament complex and consequent dislocation or fracture of the facet joints (Figs 4-39 and 4-40). A clue to this injury may be a bruise or skin injury in the vicinity of the scapula or shoulder. This injury may result from a large object landing on the patient, from a fall, or from the patient being ejected from a motor vehicle.[7,14]

Rotary atlanto-axial fixation is a relatively unusual injury first described by Fielding and Hawkins in 1977.[12] This results from disruption of the transverse ligament of the atlas and also the alar ligaments, which ordinarily prevent excessive shift of the atlas on the axis. Fielding and Hawkins describe four types of this abnormality, of which the most common involves rotary fixation without displacement of the atlas (Fig 4-41). The other varieties involve anterior or posterior displacement of the atlas.[12,17,27] These occur much less commonly. Pure rotary atlanto-axial dislocation is extremely rare. In this instance, the atlas is rotated on the axis more than 45° with resultant locking of the lateral masses of the atlas over the superior articular surfaces of the axis. This condition should not be confused with atlanto-axial rotary fixation, which is more common.

Shearing and rotational injuries are often combined, and most are associated with flexion injuries. As previously mentioned, shearing injuries result from horizontal forces. They

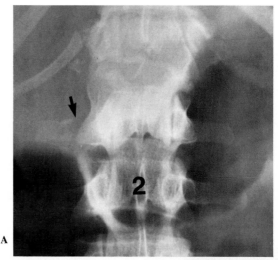

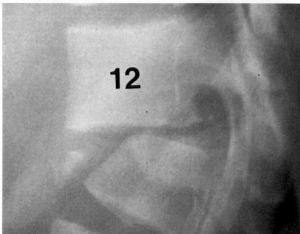

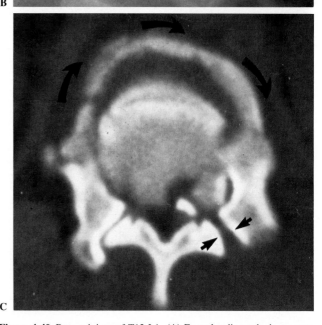

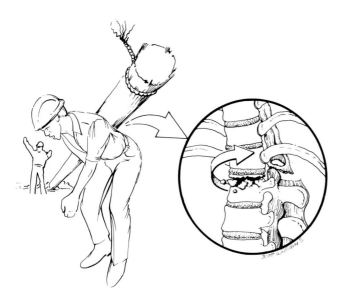

Figure 4-39 Mechanism of rotary injury (with flexion).

Figure 4-40 Rotary injury of T12-L1. **(A)** Frontal radiograph shows comminution of the body of T-12. There is a transverse process fracture of L-1 (arrow). **(B)** Lateral radiograph shows dislocation of T-12 on L-1 with compression and fragmentation of a portion of L-1. **(C)** CT scan shows fragmentation of the body of L-1 in a concentric pattern (curved arrows). Note the widening of the facet joint on the left (straight arrows).

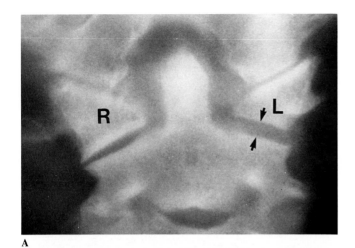

A

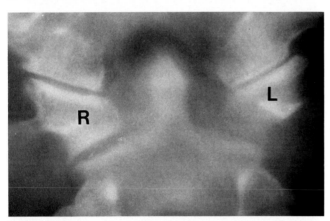

B

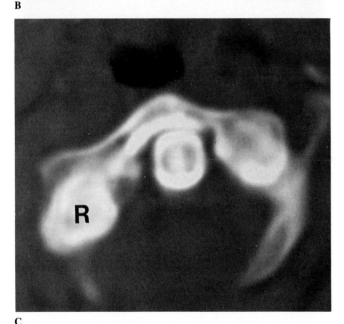

C

are extremely disruptive in nature. Rotational injuries often result from a glancing blow to the upper part of the body. They too are extremely disruptive. The fingerprints of a shearing injury are horizontal or oblique distraction and dislocation (Figs 4-37 and 4-42).[7] There are usually localized pillar and vertebral body fractures on one side.[14] If flexion is an associated component of a shearing injury, there will be angulation at the site of injury (Fig 4-43). In the lumbar region, transverse process fractures are common. The linear plane of the shearing force is usually easily identifiable on plain films (Figs 4-38 and 4-42). The shearing injuries seen at our institution were associated with lateral flexion, and all 12 occurred in the thoracolumbar region.

The fingerprints of rotational injuries in the thoracolumbar region include rotation and dislocation (Figs 4-40 and 4-44), transverse process avulsions, spinous process fractures, and findings associated with flexion injuries (Fig 4-44).[7] In the series studied at our institution, two patients had pure rotary injuries in the thoracolumbar region and nine had rotary fixations at C-2 (Fig 4-41).

Rotary fracture-dislocations may be difficult to diagnose initially because of their tendency to self-reduce after the patient is immobilized in the supine position. Malalignment of the pedicles and spinous processes on frontal radiographs is

Figure 4-41 Rotary fixation of C-1. **(A)** Frontal tomogram through the dens show asymmetry of the lateral masses of C-1. The atlanto-occipital joint on the left is more sharply defined than on the right. There is also widening of the joint space between the lateral mass on the left and the body of C-2 (arrows). **(B)** Another section farther posterior shows that the atlanto-occipital joint on the right side is sharply defined and that the one on the left is blurred. This finding indicates rotation of C-1. **(C)** CT scan shows the malalignment and malrotation.

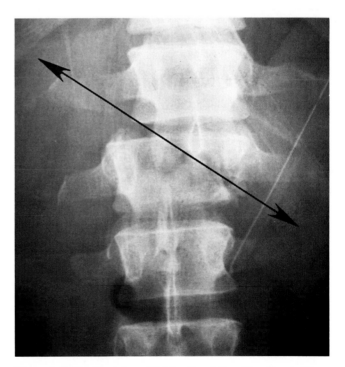

Figure 4-42 Shearing injury of L1-2 with rotation. There is an oblique fracture through the body of L-2 that extends through the pedicle on the left side. L-1 and the vertebrae above are displaced to the left. In addition, there is a fracture through the transverse process of L-1 on the right. The force vector in this instance has resulted in a nearly straight line of bony disruption (double arrow).

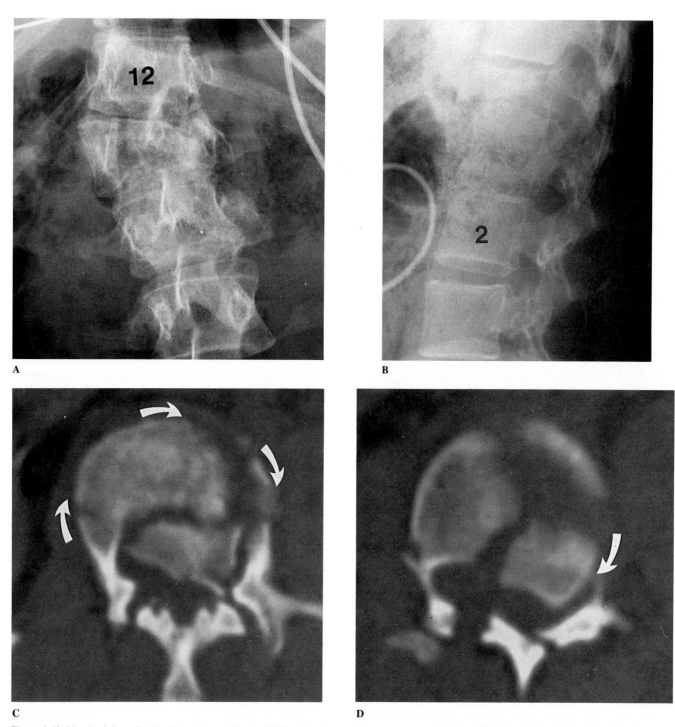

Figure 4-43 Shearing injury of L1-2 with rotation and flexion. **(A)** Frontal radiograph shows severe comminution of the body of L-1 with distortion of L-2. Note the displacement of both L-1 and L-2 in relation to the vertebrae below. **(B)** Lateral radiograph shows L-1 to be indistinct as a result of the severe comminution. **(C and D)** CT scans show severe comminution in a concentric pattern (arrows). There is widening of the facet joints. Note the bilateral fracture in **D**.

the initial clue to diagnosis (Figs 4-40 and 4-44).[14] The CT scan will show a concentric pattern to the bony fragments (Figs 4-40C, 4-43C, and 4-43D). This characteristic identifies the mechanism because the fragments are distributed along a circular pathway. Fragments resulting from a burst fracture are distributed along a horizontal plane as a result of pure linear retropulsion (Figs 4-19 and 4-20). These, combined with the additional fingerprint of a flexion injury (which is very commonly associated with thoracolumbar rotary injuries), will help determine the diagnosis.

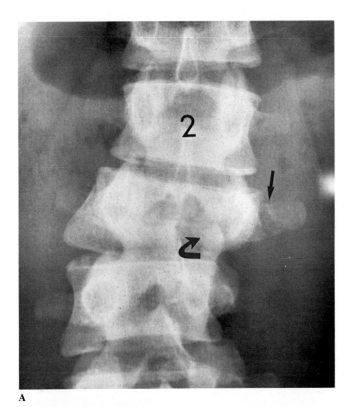

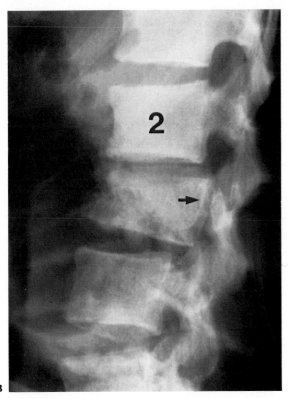

Figure 4-44 Rotary injury with burst fracture. **(A)** Frontal radiograph shows severe compression of L-3 with lateral displacement of a portion of L-3 and the vertebrae above to the left. The pattern of the fracture of the body suggests a rotary mechanism (curved arrow). Note the transverse process fracture of L-1 on the left (straight arrow). **(B)** Lateral radiograph shows posterior displacement of the body of L-3 along with further posterior displacement of the posterior vertebral body line (arrow). This is a fingerprint of the burst component.

Table 4-5 Fingerprints of Vertebral Trauma

Mechanism	Fingerprints
Flexion	1. Compression, fragmentation, burst vertebral bodies
	2. "Teardrop" fragments
	3. Wide interspinous space
	4. Anterolisthesis
	5. Disrupted posterior vertebral body line
	6. Locked facets
	7. Narrow disk space
Extension	1. Wide disk space
	2. Triangular avulsion fracture
	3. Retrolisthesis
	4. Neural arch fracture
	5. Anterolisthesis with normal interspinous space and spinolaminar line
Shearing	1. Lateral distraction
	2. Lateral dislocation
	3. Transverse process fractures
	4. Linear array of fragments
Rotation	1. Rotation
	2. Dislocation
	3. Facet and pillar fractures
	4. Transverse process fractures
	5. Circular array of fragments

Source: "Fingerprints of Vertebral Trauma—A Unifying Concept Based on Mechanisms" by RH Daffner et al in *Skeletal Radiology* (1986;15:518–525), Copyright © 1986, Springer-Verlag.

SUMMARY OF VERTEBRAL INJURY FINGERPRINTS

Table 4-5 summarizes the fingerprints of vertebral injuries.

VERTEBRAL STABILITY AND INSTABILITY

The referring physician for the spine-injured patient needs the following specific information: the presence and location of all fractures, assessment of encroachment on the vertebral canal or neural foramina by bone fragments, and assessment of vertebral stability from a radiographic standpoint. A decision about whether or not operative intervention is needed rests on the presence of encroachment and on vertebral stability. Stability of the vertebral column depends on the integrity of the major skeletal components, the intervertebral disks, the apophyseal joints, and the ligaments (Fig 4-45).[8–11,13,14,18,19]

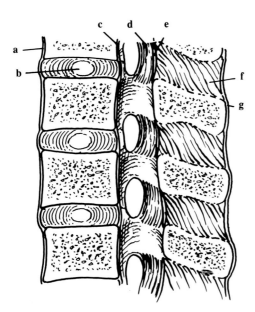

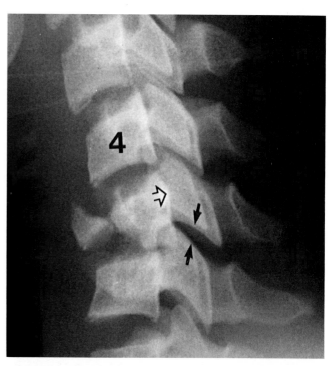

Figure 4-45 Schematic drawing of the ligamentous structures of the vertebral column in the sagittal plane. **(a)** Anterior longitudinal ligament; **(b)** nucleus pulposus; **(c)** posterior longitudinal ligament; **(d)** interfacet joint ligaments; **(e)** ligamentum flavum; **(f)** interspinous ligament; and **(g)** supraspinous ligament. *Source:* Reprinted from ''Injuries of the Thoracolumbar Vertebral Column'' by RH Daffner in *Radiology in Emergency Medicine* by MK Dalinka and JJ Kaye (Eds) with permission of Churchill Livingstone Inc., © 1984.

Figure 4-46 ''Teardrop'' fracture-dislocation of C-5 after a diving accident; unstable injury. Lateral radiograph shows the ''teardrop'' fragment of C-5. In addition, there is posterior displacement of a major portion of C-5 with buckling of the posterior vertebral body line (open arrow). Note the widening of the facet joints (closed arrows). In this instance, there are three signs that indicate instability: displacement, widened facet joints, and disrupted posterior vertebral body line.

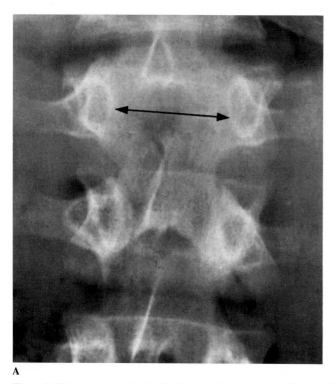

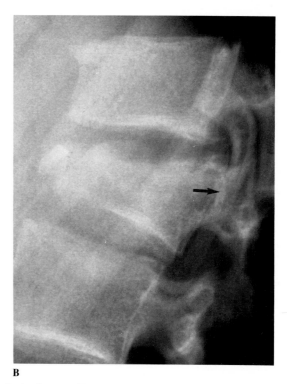

A

B

Figure 4-47 Burst fracture of L-1. **(A)** Frontal radiograph shows widening of the interpedicular distance of L-1 (double arrow). There is also loss of height of the body of L-1. **(B)** Lateral radiograph shows fragmentation of the body of L-1. There is retropulsion of a fragment of the posterior vertebral body line (arrow).

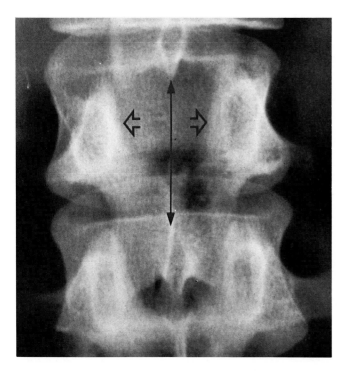

Figure 4-48 Unstable injury at T12-L1. There is widening of the interspinous space (double arrow), indicating that this patient has suffered a flexion injury. Note the "naked" facets (open arrows).

For a lesion to be considered unstable, enough damage must have occurred to allow abnormal motion at, above, or below the site of injury. Disruption of any one of the elements mentioned above may not necessarily produce an unstable injury; it is generally a combination of abnormalities that results in an unstable vertebral column.[6,7,9,10] Radiographic findings that indicate instability are displacement of vertebrae (Fig 4-46), widening of the interspinous or interlaminar spaces (Fig 4-47), widening of the apophyseal joints (Figs 4-46 and 4-48), widening and elongation of the vertebral canal manifesting as widening of the interpedicular distance in transverse and vertical planes (Figs 4-49 and 4-50), and disruption of the posterior vertebral body line (Figs 4-49 to 4-51).[7,9,10,13,14] Only one of these signs need be present to make a radiographic diagnosis of an unstable injury.

If the findings of instability are present, it is the radiologist's duty to inform the referring physician of the situation. The use of the terms "stable" and "unstable" in a radiographic report, however, is discouraged because many referring physicians may elect to treat a "mildly" unstable injury conservatively. The use of the term "unstable" in a radiographic report indicates that operative intervention is mandatory; if surgery is not performed and there is subsequent deterioration of the patient, an adversarial relationship between the radiologist and the surgeon may develop.

Unstable injuries have the potential to cause progressive neurologic deterioration, orthopaedic deformity, or death.

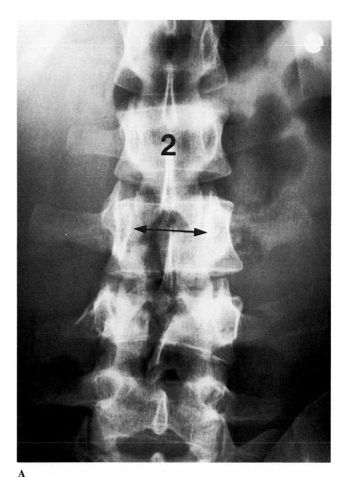

A

B

Figure 4-49 Widened interpedicular distance. The patient suffered a burst injury of L-3. **(A)** Frontal radiograph shows widening of the interpedicular distance (double arrow). **(B)** CT scan shows widening of the facet joints bilaterally (arrows) in addition to the sagittal fracture through the body of the vertebra.

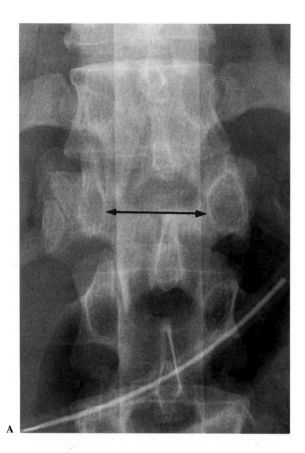

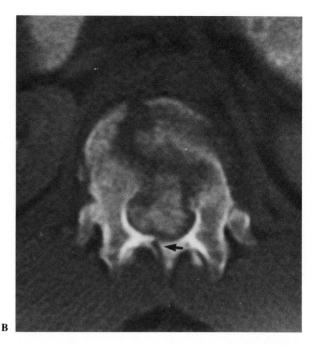

Figure 4-50 Burst fracture of T-12 with widened interpedicular space. **(A)** Frontal radiograph shows widening of the interpedicular space (double arrow). T-12 is markedly compressed. **(B)** CT scan shows comminution of the body of T-12 with a large retropulsed fragment within the vertebral canal. Fracture through the lamina on the right (arrow) allowed widening of the interpedicular distance.

The fingerprint approach to vertebral injuries can provide the physician with the necessary information to determine the management of his or her patient. Simple flexion and extension injuries are, by definition, inherently stable because the major skeletal and posterior ligamentous structures remain intact. Any injury that involves distraction or dislocation is inherently unstable because abnormal motion may occur about the site of disruption.

Denis' concept of the three-column spine helps to clarify this further.[9,10] As described earlier, Denis divides the vertebrae into three distinct functional columns. The anterior column extends from the anterior longitudinal ligament to a line drawn vertically through the center of the vertebral body in the coronal plane. The middle column begins at this line and extends to the posterior longitudinal ligament. The posterior column extends from the posterior longitudinal ligament to the supraspinous ligament (Fig 4-52). Although the major supporting structures for the vertebrae are contained within the middle and posterior columns, any disruption through two contiguous columns will result in an unstable situation. This certainly occurs with dislocation. In distraction injuries, widening of the interspinal or interlaminar distance or widening of the apophyseal joints (Figs 4-46 and 4-48) indicates the extent of the damage.

Burst fractures disrupt all three columns and thus are unstable. In addition, retropulsion of one or more central fragments usually occurs with burst injuries. This may be diagnosed on a lateral radiograph by disruption, posterior displacement, angulation, or absence of the posterior vertebral body line (Fig 4-51).[8]

The use of the fingerprint approach does have some pitfalls. The Gehweiler type IV and type V hyperextension fracture-dislocations often may be confused with unilateral articular facet lock on a lateral radiograph (Figs 4-53 and 4-54). This confusion arises from the fact that the resultant deformity produced by this injury is anteriolisthesis at the level of injury without apparent disk space widening. This lesion may be differentiated from the more common flexion injuries by the fact that the extension mechanism produces fractures of the articular pillars. The fractured pillar or pillars may often be rotated on the lateral radiograph. With this injury, however, because of the posterior fractures the spinous processes remain normally aligned, as does the spinolaminar line. The interspinous or interlaminar space is also normal (Fig 4-53). In the more common flexion injury, there is disruption of the spinolaminar line and widening of the interspinous or interlaminar space (Fig 4-54).

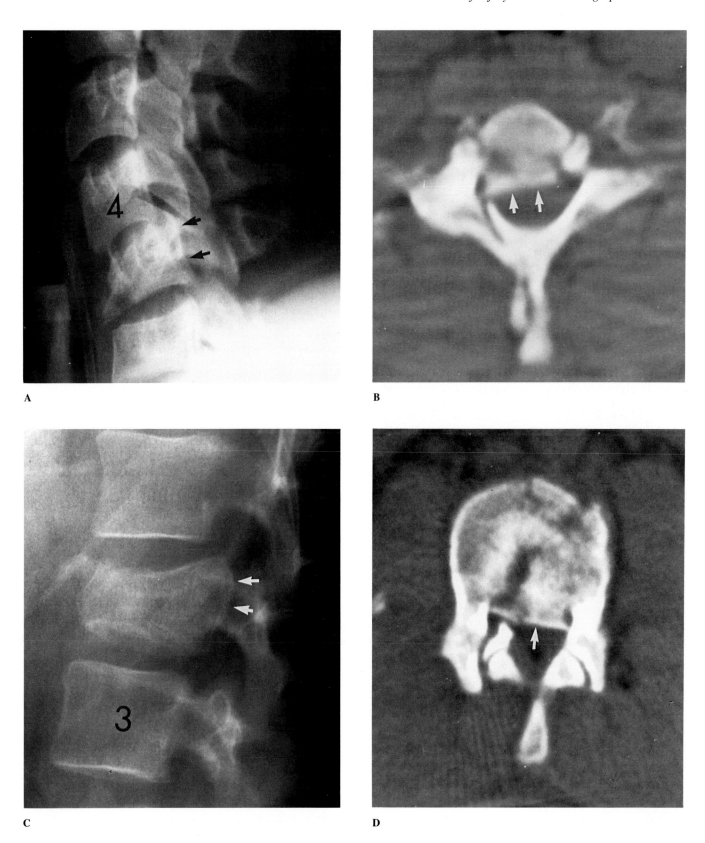

Figure 4-51 Radiographically similar burst fractures. **(A)** Lateral radiograph of a burst fracture of C-5 shows posterior displacement of the posterior vertebral body line (arrows). **(B)** CT scan of C-5 shows encroachment of this fragment of the vertebral body on the vertebral canal (arrows). **(C)** Lateral radiograph of a burst fracture of L-2 shows posterior displacement of a fragment of the body of L-2 (arrows). **(D)** CT scan of L-2 shows a central large fragment of the body of L-2 encroaching on the vertebral canal (arrow).

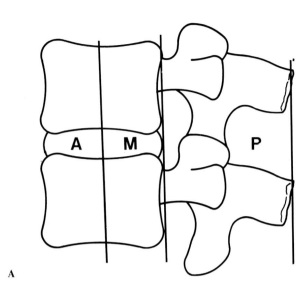

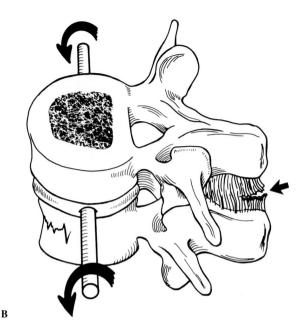

A

B

Figure 4-52 The three-column spine and mechanism of flexion injury. **(A)** Three-column spine. A, anterior column; M, middle column; P, posterior column. **(B)** Mechanism of flexion injury. Ordinary flexion produces motion about a fulcrum through the middle of the vertebral body. Excessive rotation (curved arrows) results in fractures of the anterior and superior portions of the vertebral body. As the force is continued the fracture propagates posteriorly, ultimately resulting in fragments that may be retropulsed into the vertebral canal in a burst injury. In addition, there is distraction of the posterior elements with subsequent tearing of the soft tissue structures (straight arrow). Thus a single mechanism can produce disruption of more than one vertebral compartment and produce a spectrum of injuries.

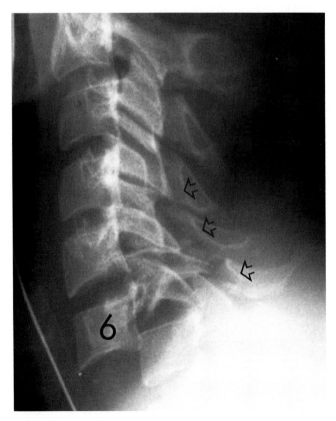

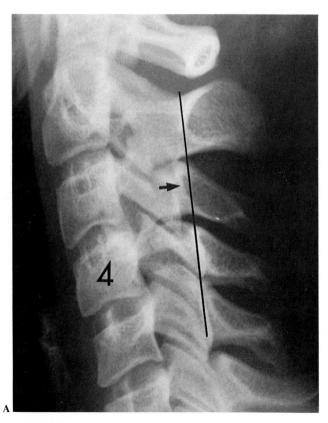

A

Figure 4-53 Hyperextension fracture-dislocation of C-6 on C-7 (Gehweiler type V). There is anterior dislocation of C-6 on C-7 with apparent locking of the facets. The spinolaminar line is intact. Compare with Fig 4-54A.

Figure 4-54 Unilateral jumped locked facets at C3-4. **(A)** Lateral radiograph shows duplication of facet shadows of C-3 and C-4. There is slight antero-listhesis at the spinolaminar line (arrow).

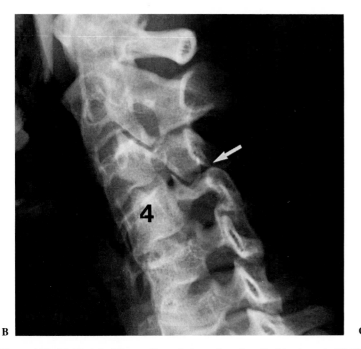

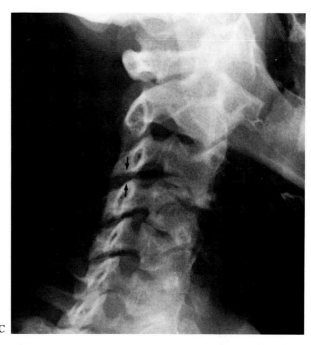

Figure 4-54 (B) The left oblique radiograph shows the point of locking (arrow). **(C)** The right oblique radiograph shows normal alignment of the articular pillars. There is widening of the facet joint of C3-4 (arrows).

REFERENCES

1. Atlas SW, Regenbogen V, Rogers LF, et al: The radiographic characterization of burst fractures of the spine. *AJR* 1986;147:575–582.

2. Burke DC: Hyperextension injuries of the spine. *J Bone Joint Surg* 1971;53B:3–12.

3. Calenoff L, Chessare JW, Rogers LF, et al: Multiple level spinal injuries: Importance of early recognition. *AJR* 1978;130:665–669.

4. Chance GQ: Note on a type of flexion fracture of the spine. *Br J Radiol* 1948;21:452–453.

5. Cintron E, Gilula LA, Murphy WA, et al: The widened disk space: A sign of cervical hyperextension injury. *Radiology* 1981;141:639–644.

6. Clark WM, Gehweiler JA, Laib R: Twelve significant signs of cervical spine trauma. *Skeletal Radiol* 1979;3:201–205.

7. Daffner RH, Deeb ZL, Rothfus WE: "Fingerprints" of vertebral trauma—A unifying concept based on mechanisms. *Skeletal Radiol* 1986; 15:518–525.

8. Daffner RH, Deeb ZL, Rothfus WE: The posterior vertebral body line: Importance in the detection of burst fractures. *AJR* 1987;148:93–96.

9. Denis F: The three-column spine and its significance in the classification of acute thoracolumbar spinal injuries. *Spine* 1983;8:817–831.

10. Denis F: Spinal instability as defined by the three-column spine concept in acute spinal trauma. *Clin Orthop* 1984;189:65–76.

11. Ferguson RL, Allen BL Jr: A mechanistic classification of thoracolumbar spine fractures. *Clin Orthop* 1984;189:77–88.

12. Fielding JW, Hawkins RJ: Atlanto-axial rotatory fixation: Fixed rotatory subluxation of the atlanto-axial joint. *J Bone Joint Surg* 1977; 59A:37–44.

13. Gehweiler JA Jr, Daffner RH, Osborne RL Jr: Relevant signs of stable and unstable thoracolumbar vertebral column trauma. *Skeletal Radiol* 1981; 7:179–183.

14. Gehweiler JA Jr, Osborne RL Jr, Becker RF: *The Radiology of Vertebral Trauma.* Philadelphia, WB Saunders, 1980.

15. Guerra J Jr, Garfin SR, Resnick D: Vertebral burst fractures: CT analysis of the retropulsed fragment. *Radiology* 1984;153:769–772.

16. Holdsworth FW: Review article: Fractures, dislocations, and fracture-dislocations of the spine. *J Bone Joint Surg* 1970;52A:1534–1551.

17. Jacobson G, Alder DC: Examination of the atlanto-axial joint following injury with particular emphasis on rotational subluxation. *AJR* 1956; 76:1081–1094.

18. Mazur JM, Stauffer ESP: Unrecognized spinal instability associated with seemingly "simple" cervical compression fractures. *Spine* 1983; 8:687–692.

19. McAfee PC, Yuan HA, Lasda NA: The unstable burst fracture. *Spine* 1983;7:365–373.

20. Roaf R: A study of the mechanics of spinal injuries. *J Bone Joint Surg* 1960;42B:810–823.

21. Roaf R: International classification of spinal injuries. *Paraplegia* 1972; 10:78–84.

22. Schneider RC, Livingston KE, Cave AJE, et al: "Hangman's fracture" of the cervical spine. *J Neurosurg* 1965;22:141–154.

23. Seljeskog EL, Chous SN: Spectrum of the hangman's fracture. *J Neurosurg* 1976;3:45–48.

24. Smith WS, Kaufer H: Patterns and mechanisms of lumbar injuries associated with lap seatbelts. *J Bone Joint Surg* 1969;51A:239–254.

25. Whitley JE, Forsyth HF: The classification of cervical spine injuries. *AJR* 1960;83:633–644.

26. Woodruff FP, Dewing SB: Fracture of the cervical spine in patients with ankylosing spondylitis. *Radiology* 1963;80:17–21.

27. Wortzman G, Dewar FP: Rotary fixation of the atlantoaxial joint: Rotational atlantoaxial subluxation. *Radiology* 1968;90:479–487.

Chapter 5

ABCS of Radiologic Interpretation of Vertebral Trauma

The initial assessment of any patient with suspected vertebral trauma should be by plain film radiography. It is from the plain radiographs that the main diagnosis may be made. The use of computed tomography (CT), polydirectional tomography (PT), or magnetic resonance imaging (MRI) should be directed toward confirming the initial diagnosis established from the plain radiographs and to delineate the full extent of injury by demonstrating additional fractures not shown on plain films. The interpretation of any radiographic examination demands that a logical system be followed, such as the "ABCS" of evaluating the vertebral column:

A—Alignment and anatomy
B—Bony integrity
C—Cartilage (joint) spaces
S— Soft tissues

This chapter presents a detailed discussion of the various radiographic findings given in the preceding chapters and shows how they are integrated into the overall diagnosis of traumatic lesions of the vertebral column.

ABNORMALITIES OF ALIGNMENT AND ANATOMY

Chapter 2 discussed the detailed anatomy of the bones, joints, and ligaments of the vertebral column. A thorough knowledge of normal anatomy and the variants of that anatomy is prerequisite for interpretation of vertebral radiographs.

Normal alignment may be determined on all radiographs. Of all the views employed in the evaluation of the vertebral column, the lateral view is the most important for assessing alignment. This is true throughout the vertebral column.

Normal markers of alignment on the lateral view include the anterior and posterior margins of the vertebral bodies, the spinolaminar line, the articular pillars and their facet joints, and the interspinous or interlaminar distance (Fig 5-1). Under normal circumstances, a line drawn along the anterior or posterior margins of the vertebral bodies should be smooth and uninterrupted. A notable exception is in the cervical column of children, in whom pseudosubluxation occurs because of the disparate growth rates of the various portions of the vertebral column (Fig 5-2).[5,12,18] Similarly, a line connecting the junction of the laminae with the spinous processes (the spinolaminar line or the arch canal line) should be smooth and unbroken. Note that even with the pseudosubluxation of childhood, there are no disruptions of the spinolaminar line (Fig 5-2). On a perfectly centered lateral film, the articular pillars in the cervical region and the articular processes in the thoracic and lumbar regions should be symmetric and should appear as single shadows.

Minor degrees of rotation (as evidenced by malalignment of the mandibular shadow in the cervical region) may result in double facet shadows. This usually does not present a diag-

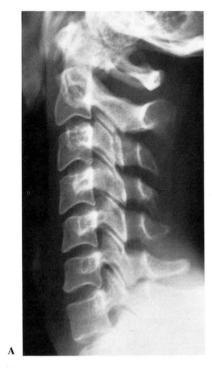

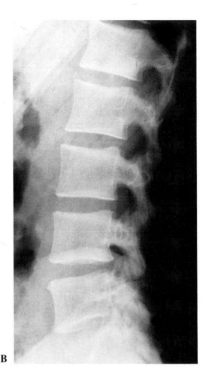

A

B

Figure 5-1 (**A**) Normal lateral cervical vertebral column. Note the uniform alignment of the anterior and posterior margins of the vertebral bodies. The spinolaminar line is also smooth and unbroken. The interspinous and interlaminar spaces are uniform, and the facet joints appear to be symmetric. (**B**) Normal lateral lumbar column. The anterior and posterior margins of the vertebral bodies form a smooth, uninterrupted line. There is a normal, mildly lordotic curve to the lumbar column.

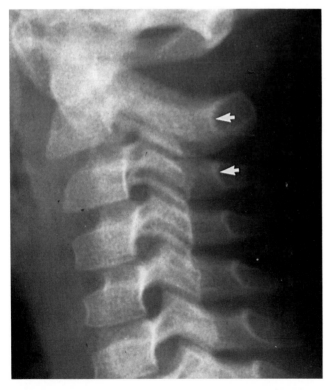

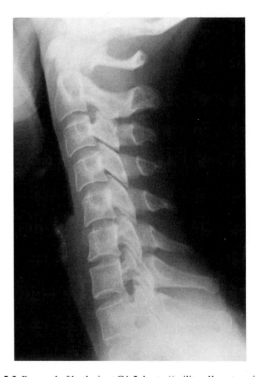

Figure 5-2 Pseudosubluxation of C-2 on C-3 in a young child. There is apparent anterolisthesis of C-2 on C-3 due to a disparity of growth rates between these two vertebrae. The spinolaminar line (arrows) is uniform.

Figure 5-3 Reversal of lordosis at C4-5 due to ''military'' posture, in which the patient's chin is tucked back. There are no abnormalities of the spinolaminar line, facet joints, or soft tissues. If a question remains about occult injury in such a patient, lateral erect flexion and extension views should be obtained.

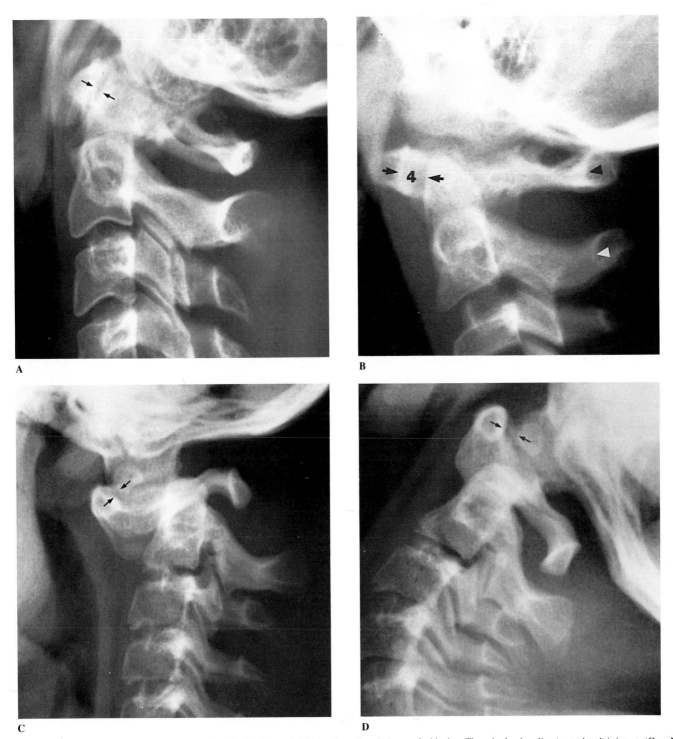

Figure 5-4 Predental space (arrows). (**A**) Normal adult. (**B**) Normal child in whom there is 4 mm of widening. The spinolaminar line (arrowhead) is intact. (**C and D**) Atlanto-axial dislocation in a patient with os odontoideum. Flexion (**C**) and extension (**D**) views show the extent of motion. The predental space is widened in each case.

nostic problem. The space between the spinous processes at the level of the spinolaminar line or between the laminae themselves (the interspinous space and the interlaminar space, respectively) should be symmetric and should not vary by more than 2 mm from one level to the next. In the cervical region, straightening of the neck resulting from the "military" posture usually does not result in dramatic changes in these spaces (Fig 5-3).[13]

In the craniocervical region (Fig 5-4), there are special considerations related to the different anatomy.[10,12,14,17,28]

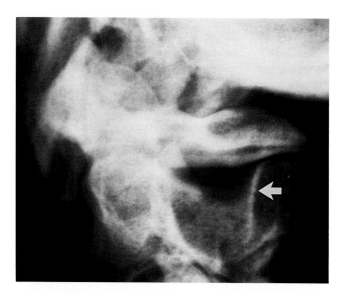

Figure 5-5 Failure of fusion of the posterior arch of C-1. The dense white arch canal line at C-2 (arrow) is absent at C-1, indicating the anomaly.

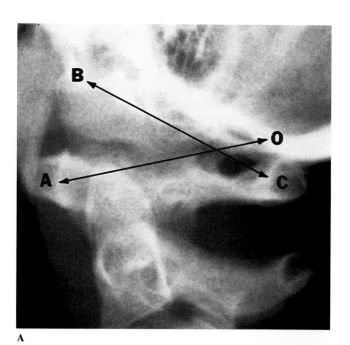

A

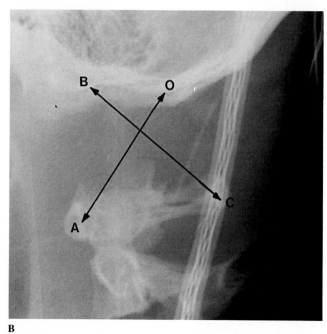

B

Figure 5-6 Powers' ratio. (**A**) Lines are drawn from the basion to the midpoint of the posterior arch of C-1 (B–C) and from the opisthion to the posterior surface of the anterior arch of the atlas (O–A). Here the ratio B–C:O–A is less than 1, which is normal. (**B**) Atlanto-occipital dislocation. The ratio B–C:O–A is 1.2 in this very obvious dislocation.

The anterior arch of the atlas bears a constant relationship to the dens. The predental space between these structures should be no greater than 3 mm in an adult and 5 mm in a child. The posterior arches of the atlas merge in the midline to form the posterior tubercle. This creates a dense shadow that aligns with the spinolaminar line. In individuals in whom fusion has not occurred in the posterior arch of the atlas, this dense line is absent. Alignment will then depend on assessment of the anterior structures (Fig 5-5).

The relationship between the base of the skull and the atlas may be assessed by means of the Powers' ratio,[13,26] which is determined by measuring the distances from four points (Fig 5-6). The first line is drawn from the basion to the midpoint of the arch canal line on the posterior arch of the atlas (line B–C). The second line is drawn from the opisthion to the midpoint of the posterior surface of the anterior arch of the atlas (line O–A). Under normal circumstances, the ratio B–C:O–A should be less than 1.[13,26]

An alternative method was described by Lee and associates (Fig 5-7).[20] In this method, a line (the descending limb) is drawn between the clivus or basion to the midpoint of the spinolaminar line of C-2. A second line (the ascending limb) is drawn from the posteroinferior corner of the body of C-2 to the opisthion. Under normal circumstances, the descending limb should touch the dens or be within 5 mm of it. The ascending limb should pass through the spinolaminar line of C-1.

On the frontal views (Fig 5-8), alignment may be assessed by looking at the lateral margins of the vertebrae, the pedicles, the spinous processes, the uncinate processes in the cervical region, and the facet joints in the thoracic and lumbar regions.[13] Under normal circumstances, lines drawn along each of these margins should be straight and uninterrupted. There should be less than 2 mm difference from one level to the next. In the thoracic and lumbar regions, the difference in the transverse distance between the pedicles (interpedicular distance) should be less than 2 mm from level to level. Any deviation greater than 2 mm should be considered abnormal

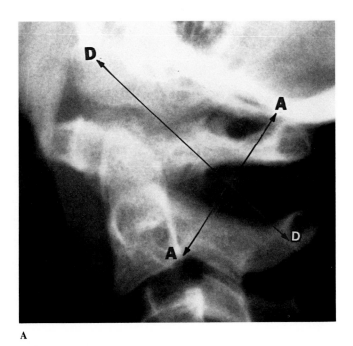

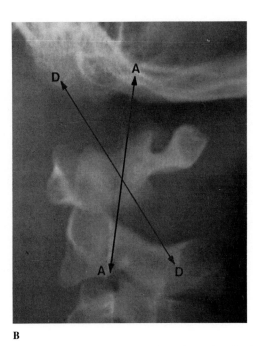

A   B

Figure 5-7 Lee method of assessing atlanto-occipital relationships. (**A**) Normal child. The descending limb (D–D) extends from the basion to the midpoint of the posterior arch of the axis. The ascending limb (A–A) extends from the posteroinferior corner of the body of C-2 to the opisthion. In this instance, the measurements were normal and magnification factors were considered. (**B**) Atlanto-occipital dislocation. There is gross disruption of the Lee lines in this very obvious dislocation. This method is of great value in more subtle cases.

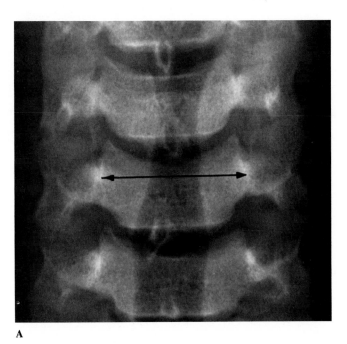

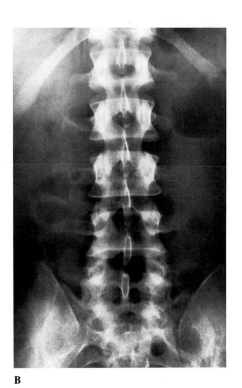

A   B

Figure 5-8 Normal frontal views. (**A**) Cervical region. The spinous processes should be in normal alignment, and the distance between them should be uniform. The spaces between the articular pillars should also be uniform, and the distance between pedicles (double arrow) should be uniform from level to level. (**B**) Lumbar region. The same parameters for the cervical region hold true in the lumbar and thoracic regions.

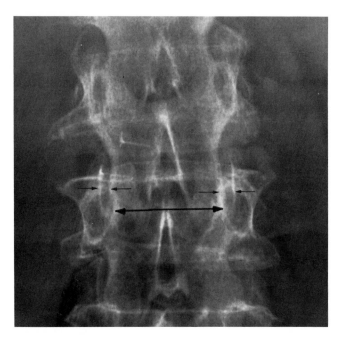

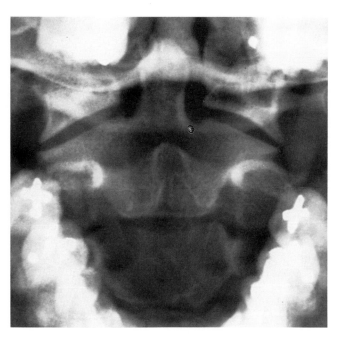

Figure 5-9 Widened interpedicular distance of L-3 as a result of a burst fracture. Compare the interpedicular distance of L-3 (double arrow) with that of its mates. There is also widening of the facet joints at L-3 (small arrows).

Figure 5-10 Normal atlanto-axial view. The lateral alignment between the lateral mass of C-1 and the body of C-2 should be uniform. Up to 2 mm of unilateral or bilateral lateral offset is allowed in the presence of a congenital anomaly of C-1. Minor differences in the width of the space between the dens and the lateral masses of C-1 may occur with rotation.

(Fig 5-9). Similarly, the difference in the vertical interpedicular distances should be symmetric and less than 2 mm at each level. When the spinous processes are used to assess alignment, rotation off the midline as well as widening of the interspinous space should be noted.[7,8,11,13,23,24] The frontal view is ideal for this purpose.

In the cranioverbral region, there are, as on the lateral view, additional considerations. Under normal circumstances, the inion of the occipital bone (internal occipital protuberance), the dens, and the spinous processes of C-2 and C-3 should align.[13] Minor degrees of rotation result in differences in the distance between the dens and the lateral masses of C-1. When this is encountered, it is important to check the other alignment points in this area to determine whether the abnormality is due to rotation rather than to ligamentous disruption.

The lateral masses of C-1 should normally align with the body and lateral aspect of C-2 (Fig 5-10). In children, there may be up to 3 mm of disparity in the lateral atlanto-axial border due to differences in growth rate between the two bones (Fig 5-11).[5,12,18,30] In adults, up to 2 mm of lateral atlanto-axial overlap may be considered normal if the patient has some form of anomaly of C-1 (Fig 5-12).[12] Malalignment by more than 3 mm in children or adults is usually encountered in a Jefferson-type burst fracture (Fig 5-13).[12,13,19,20]

The oblique views may also be used to assess alignment (Fig 5-14). The anterior and posterior vertebral body margin should normally align. A line drawn along the anterior or posterior margins of the pedicles should be smooth and uninterrupted, as should a line drawn across the laminae. In addition the facet joints should be symmetric in their alignment, in much the same way that shingling overlaps on a roof (imbrication).[13] In the cervical region, the intervertebral foramina and their margins should be symmetric.

Abnormalities of alignment may be easily detected because of the disruptions they produce in the structures or lines described above. The most common abnormality is anterolisthesis, which is often seen in flexion injuries (Figs 5-15 and 5-16).[8] As mentioned in Chapter 4, the findings often indicate combined abnormalities, and anterolisthesis is usually accompanied by widening of the interspinous or interlaminar space and widening of the facet joints (Figs 5-15 to 5-17). For example, in a patient with unilateral facet lock (Fig 5-18), in addition to anterolisthesis the spinous process on the frontal film is rotated toward the side of the locked facet.[4,7,8,13] The lateral film in such a patient demonstrates, in addition to the anterolisthesis, duplication of the facet shadows above the level of lock. Below the level of lock, there is the normal overlap of both facet shadows. Above this level,

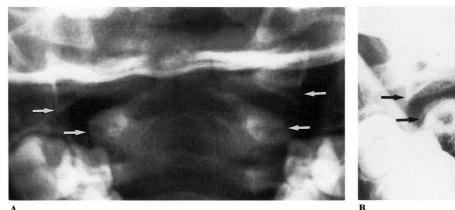

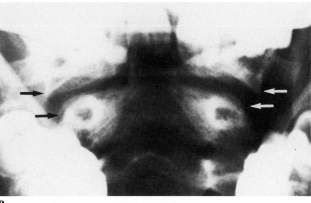

Figure 5-11 (**A and B**) Atlanto-axial malalignment in children. Radiographs of two different children show malalignment of the lateral masses of C-1 with respect to the body of C-2 (arrows). Often the difference may be striking because of differences in the growth rate between the two bones. As the child grows, the relationship becomes normal.

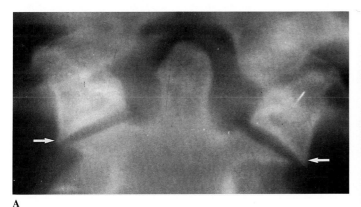

Figure 5-12 Bilateral lateral atlanto-axial offset in a patient in whom the posterior arch of C-1 did not fuse. (**A**) Frontal tomogram shows the overhang of the lateral masses of C-1 on the body of C-2 (arrows). (**B**) Lateral radiograph shows absence of the arch canal line at C-1. *Source:* Reprinted with permission from "Malformations of the Atlas Vertebra Simulating the Jefferson Fracture" by JA Gehweiler Jr, RH Daffner, and L Roberts Jr in *American Journal of Roentgenology* (1983;140:1083–1086), Copyright © 1983, American Roentgen Ray Society.

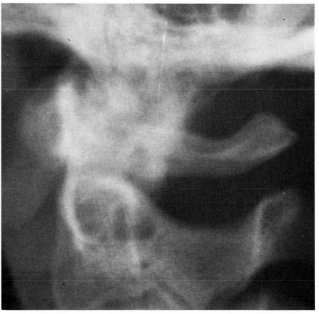

two distinct facet shadows are seen (Figs 5-18 and 5-19). The transition is abrupt, which serves to differentiate this condition from simple positional rotation.

Additional abnormalities may be detected by observing the facet images and spinolaminar line. If a patient has a dislocation with locking of the facets, and if the spinolaminar line is in its normal position, then bilateral fractures are present in either the pedicles or laminae (Fig 5-20). It is easy to understand this finding because the spinolaminar line would be disrupted if an intact posterior arch were present.

Degenerative anterolisthesis or retrolisthesis may cause diagnostic difficulty in a traumatized patient. Lee and associates have shown that in degenerative slippage the articular facets are "ground down" with narrowing of the facet joint space. In traumatic luxation, the articular facets are either normal or fractured and the facet joint spaces are abnormally widened (Figs 5-16 and 5-17).[21]

Lateral flexion injuries in the cervical region may result in an isolated crush fracture to an articular pillar. This unusual injury may be detected by observing rotation of the pillar

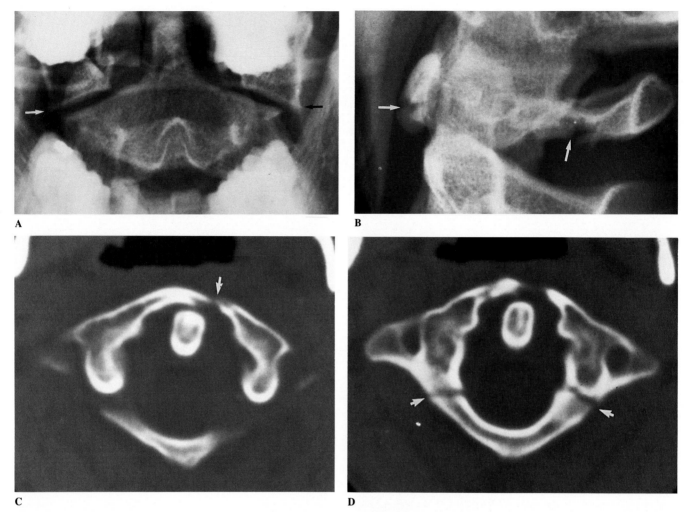

A   B

C   D

Figure 5-13 Jefferson fracture. (**A**) Open-mouth atlanto-axial view shows bilateral lateral atlanto-axial malalignment (arrows). (**B**) Lateral radiograph shows fractures in both the anterior and posterior arches of C-1 (arrows). (**C and D**) CT scans show the anterior (**C**) and posterior (**D**) arch fractures (arrows).

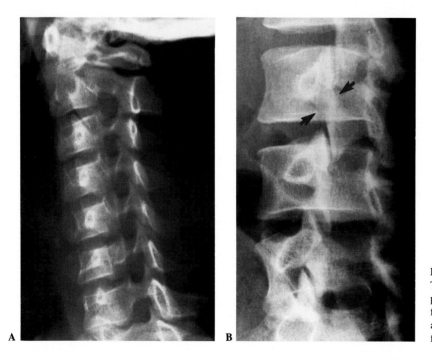

A   B

Figure 5-14 Normal oblique views. (**A**) Cervical region. There is normal alignment of the vertebral bodies, articular pillars, and transverse process images. The intervertebral foramina are uniform. (**B**) Lumbar region. There is normal alignment of the vertebral bodies, pedicles, and articular facets. The pars interarticularis (arrows) is uniform.

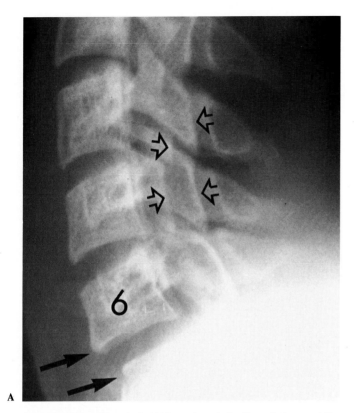

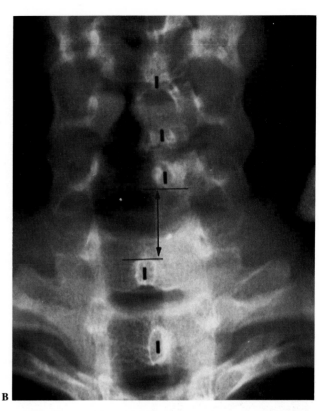

Figure 5-15 Unilateral facet lock. (**A**) Lateral cervical radiograph shows malalignment of C-6 on C-7. Note the anterolisthesis at that level (solid arrows). The point of locking is obscured by the patient's heavy shoulders. There is, however, duplication of the articular pillar images above C-6 (open arrows). (**B**) Frontal radiograph shows malalignment of the spinous processes (vertical dashes). There is also widening of the interspinous space (double arrow).

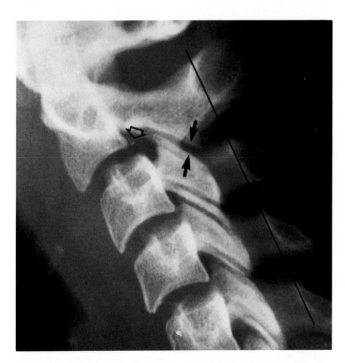

Figure 5-16 Flexion sprain at C2-3 with displacement. There is malalignment of the spinolaminar line (solid line) and widening of the facet joints of C2-3 (solid arrows). There is an avulsion of a small sliver of bone from the posteroinferior aspect of C-2 (open arrow). Ligamentous damage has resulted in slight anterolisthesis of C-2 on C-3.

images on lateral and oblique radiographs (Fig 5-21).[13,27] The only way for this rotation to have occurred is if both the pedicle and lamina on the same side were fractured.

Acute kyphotic angulation and loss of lordosis are additional findings that may indicate underlying injury. A common injury is hyperflexion sprain, in which the posterior ligaments are ruptured.[13] In these individuals, a supine lateral radiograph may often appear normal. In the erect position, however, the weight of the head will produce acute kyphotic angulation with widening of the interspinous or interlaminar space (Fig 5-22). This is to be differentiated from positional loss of lordosis or lordosis due to simple muscle spasm without ligamentous injury. In these cases, there is an abnormal curvature to the spine but no disruption in the spinolaminar line or widening between spinous processes (Fig 5-23). Similarly, loss of lordosis in the lumbar area may be the result of muscle spasm rather than underlying injury; in most instances, if there is an injury there are usually other radiographic manifestations. Finally, torticollis in the neck produces an alignment abnormality, but this is a nonspecific sign and usually is the result of muscle spasm.

Table 5-1 (see p. 112) summarizes alignment abnormalities.

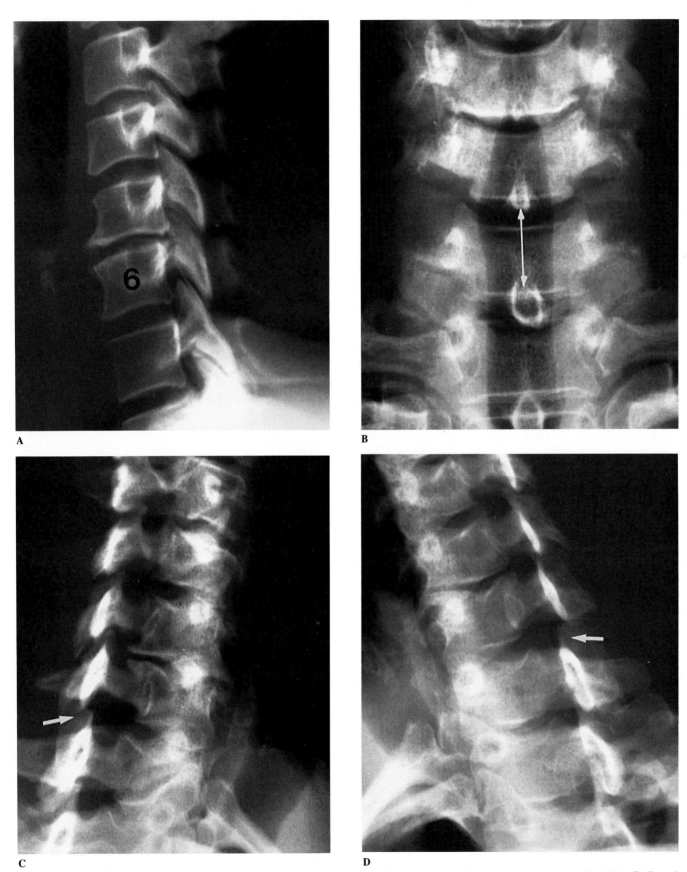

A

B

C

D

Figure 5-17 Flexion sprain. (**A**) A single lateral view shows degenerative changes at C5-6. No other significant abnormalities can be identified. (**B**) Frontal radiograph shows widening of the interspinous space of C6-7 (double arrow). (**C and D**) Oblique views show widening of the facet joints at C6-7 bilaterally (arrows). These findings, although subtle, represent significant ligamentous injury in this patient.

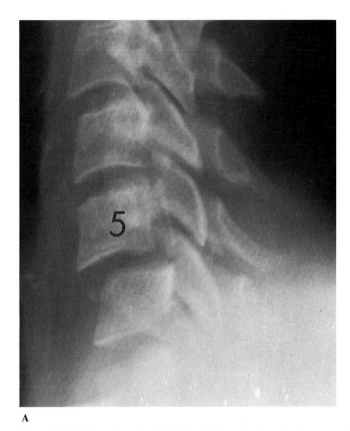

A

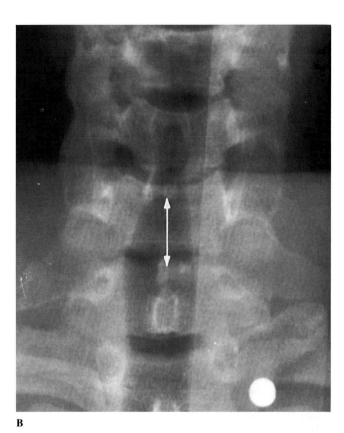

B

Figure 5-18 Unilateral facet lock of C5-6. (**A**) Lateral radiograph shows anterolisthesis of C-5 on C-6. (**B**) Frontal radiograph shows widening of the interspinous space between C-5 and C-6 (double arrow). Note the subtle shift of the spinous processes of C-5 and above to the right side, indicating that this is the side of locking.

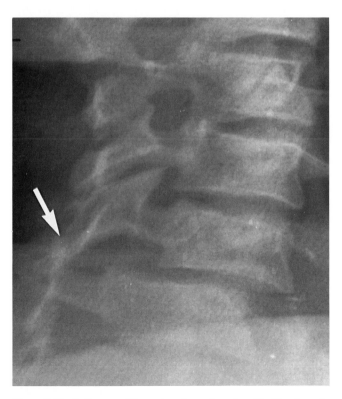

Figure 5-18 (**C**) Trauma oblique view shows the point of locking (arrow).

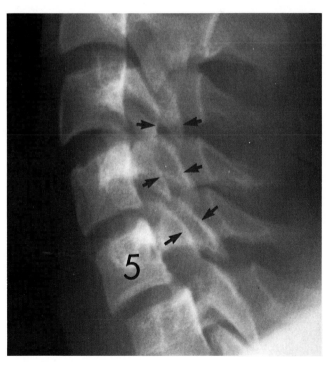

Figure 5-19 Unilateral facet lock. There is anterolisthesis of C-5 on C-6. Note the single articular pillar image of C-6. All the images above C-6 are duplicated (arrows).

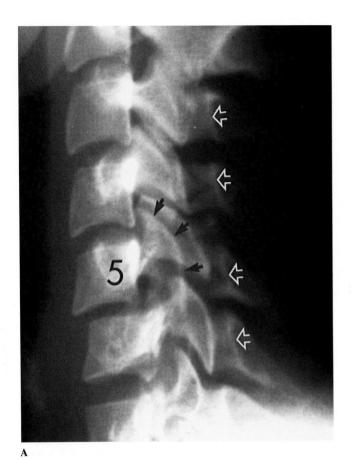

A

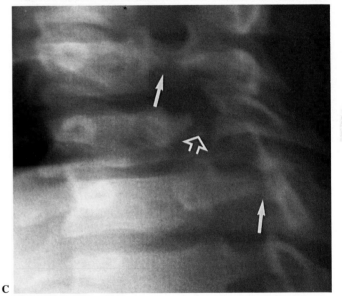

B

C

Figure 5-20 Extension fracture–dislocation of C5-6 (Gehweiler type IV). (**A**) Lateral radiograph shows anterolisthesis of the body of C-5 on C-6. The spinolaminar line (open arrows) remains intact. There is duplication of a pillar image of C-5, indicating a free-floating pillar (solid arrows). (**B and C**) Trauma oblique views show bilateral pedicle fractures of C-5 (open arrows). In addition, there are fractures of the pedicles of C-4 and C-6 on the left (solid arrows in **C**).

ABNORMALITIES IN BONY INTEGRITY

Any disruption in the bone indicates a fracture. There are subtle findings that can aid in diagnosis, however. Four of these signs are disruption of the posterior vertebral body line, wide interpedicular distance, disruption in the C-2 body ring, and disruption of the arcuate lines of the sacrum.

As mentioned in Chapter 2, the posterior border of the vertebral body casts a single vertical line or shadow in the cervical region (Fig 5-24A) and a single vertical line with central interruption in the thoracic and lumbar regions (Fig 5-24B).[9] This central interruption is the site of the basivertebral vein as it traverses the vertebral body. Any other

interruption, displacement, or angulation of this line or absence of the line should be considered an abnormal finding. This is especially important in individuals who have suffered flexion injuries; any of these findings is indicative of a burst fracture. Burst fractures usually produce retropulsion of one or more large fragments from the posterior aspect of the vertebral body (Figs 5-25 to 5-28). Disruption of the posterior vertebral body line on a plain film indicates the extent of injury and, when combined with additional alignment abnormalities, is an indicator of an unstable injury.[3,9,11,13]

Burst injuries tend to explode the vertebral body and separate it from its posterior elements. One of these manifestations, particularly in the thoracolumbar region, is widening of

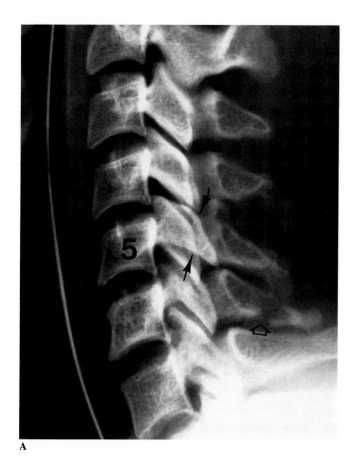

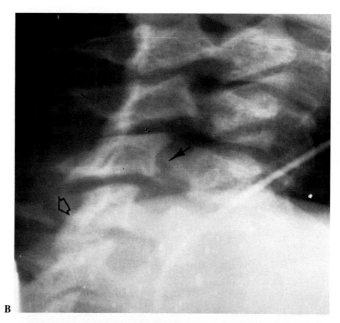

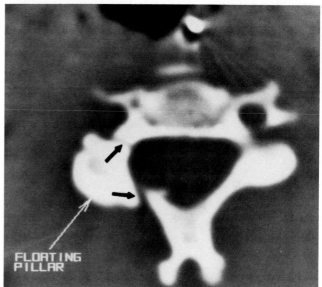

Figure 5-21 Floating pillar. **(A)** Lateral radiograph shows normal alignment of all elements, with the exception of a duplicate pillar image of C-5 (solid arrows). There is a spinous process fracture of C-6 (open arrow). **(B)** Trauma oblique view shows a fracture through the pillar of C-5 on the right side (solid arrow). The spinous process fracture of C-6 can also be seen (open arrow). Note the rotation of the pillar of C-5. **(C)** CT scan shows asymmetry of the pillars of C-5 as a result of the fractures of the lamina and pedicle on the right side (black arrows). The pillar of C-5 on the right is floating.

the transverse interpedicular distance (Figs 5-29 and 5-30). This may be easily discerned by measuring the distance between the pedicles on frontal radiographs. When present, the widening also indicates posterior arch disruption. In most cases there are additional findings indicative of burst injury, including widening of the interspinous distance, naked facets, comminution of the vertebral body, and, as mentioned above, disruption of the posterior vertebral body line.[8,9,11,13]

On a lateral radiograph of C-2 there is a ringlike density at the base of the dens. Harris and associates described this finding as a composite of shadows (Fig 5-31).[15] By using

dried specimens and wires, they were able to demonstrate that the superior arc of the ring is due to the superior articulating facet that is obliquely oriented with regard to the central beam. The anterior and posterior arcs of the ring are formed by the junction points of the body of the axis and the contiguous structures. The inferior arc of the ring is produced by the thin transverse process superimposed on the foramen transversarium. The dens does not contribute to the ring. This ring sign is extremely useful in identifying patients with the so-called type III odontoid fracture, which is actually a fracture of the body of C-2 (Figs 5-32 and 5-33).[1,2,15] These fractures are

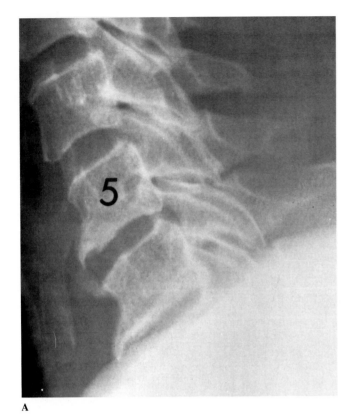

A

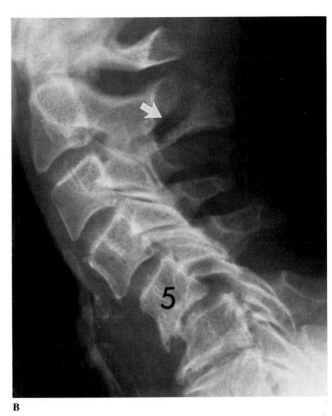

B

Figure 5-22 Flexion sprain of C-5. (**A**) Lateral supine radiograph with the patient in a restraining collar shows normal vertebral alignment. There are mild degenerative changes. (**B**) Upright radiograph obtained after removal of the collar shows marked anterolisthesis of C-5 on C-6, widening of the interspinous space, and luxation of the facet joints. In addition, there is a fracture of the spinous process of C-2 (arrow) that was not apparent on the initial supine radiograph. This case illustrates the need to obtain upright lateral radiographs before the patient is discharged.

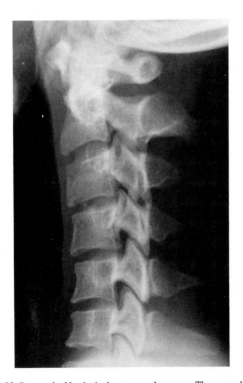

Figure 5-23 Reversal of lordosis due to muscle spasm. The normal lordotic curve is lost. There is no malalignment in this otherwise normal lateral cervical column.

Table 5-1 Alignment Abnormalities

Disruption of anterior or posterior veterbral body lines
Disruption of spinolaminar line
Jumped and locked facets
Rotation of spinous process
Widening of interpedicular space
Widening of predental space
Acute kyphotic angulation
Loss of lordosis
Torticollis

---

difficult to diagnose on plain films because there is seldom any displacement of the bony fragments.

Recently, Smoker and Dolan[29] described another sign of a fracture of the body of C-2. This sign results from the shift of fracture fragments to produce apparent widening of the body of C-2 in relation to C-3. They termed this the "fat" C-2 sign. It is a valuable sign for the identification of subtle C-2 fractures (Fig 5-33). A CT scan will generally confirm the fracture.

(text continues on p. 117)

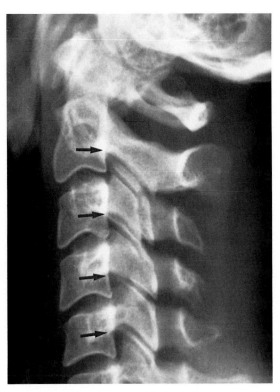

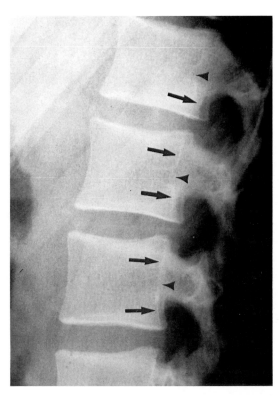

Figure 5-24 Normal posterior vertebral body lines (arrows): (**A**) cervical region, (**B**) lumbar region. In the cervical region, these lines are unbroken. In the thoracolumbar region, they may be interrupted by nutrient foramina (arrowheads in **B**).

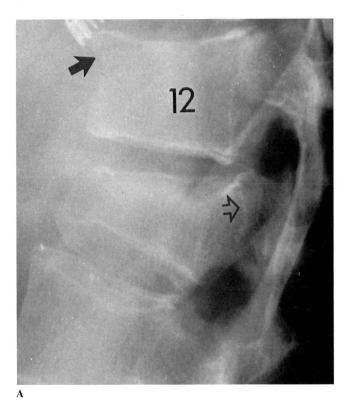

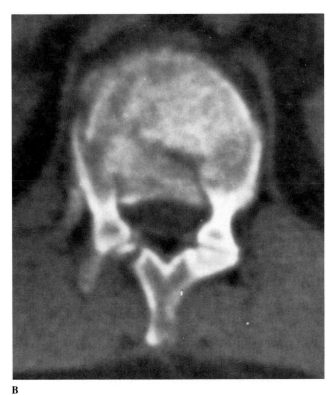

A   **B**

Figure 5-25 Burst fracture of L-1. (**A**) Lateral radiograph shows loss of height of the body of L-1. A portion of the posterior vertebral body line has been displaced superiorly (open arrow). There is also a simple compression fracture of the anterosuperior lip of T-12 (solid arrow). (**B**) CT scan through the upper portion of the body of L-1 shows a large intracanalicular fragment that has been displaced posteriorly. This accounts for the abnormal appearance of the posterior vertebral body line.

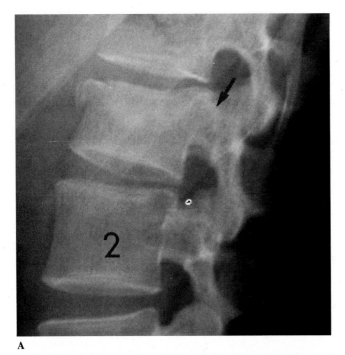

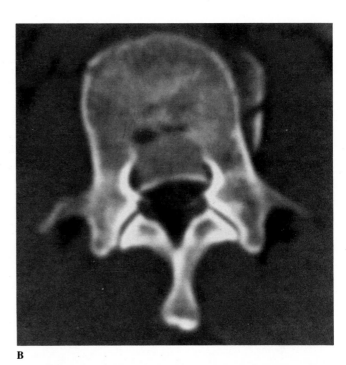

A   B

Figure 5-26 Burst fracture of L-1 with displacement of the posterior vertebral body line. (**A**) There is loss of height of the body of L-1 with a compression fracture of the anterosuperior lip of that vertebra. The superior aspect of the posterior vertebral body line has been displaced (arrow). This indicates a burst fracture. (**B**) CT scan through the region shows the free fragment of bone that has been displaced posteriorly to encroach on the vertebral canal. This accounts for the abnormal posterior vertebral body line seen in **A**. *Source:* Reprinted with permission from ''The Posterior Vertebral Body Line: Importance in the Detection of Burst Fractures'' by RH Daffner, ZL Deeb, and WE Rothfus in *American Journal of Roentgenology* (1987;148:93–96), Copyright © 1987, American Roentgen Ray Society.

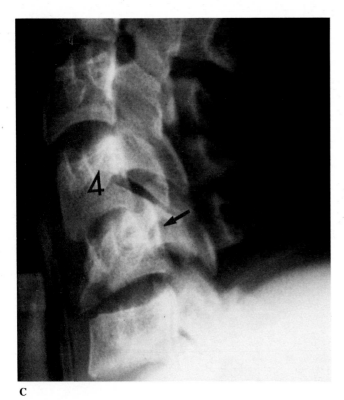

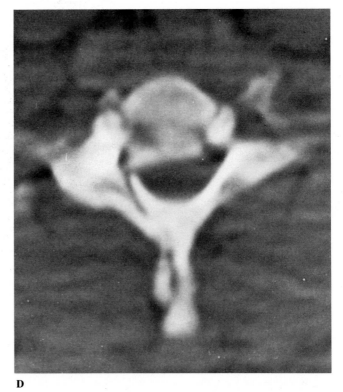

C   D

Figure 5-27 Cervical burst fracture of C-5. (**A**) Lateral radiograph shows posterior displacement of a bony fragment into the vertebral canal (arrow). There is severe comminution of the body of C-5 and anterolisthesis of C-4 on C-5. (**B**) CT scan through the region shows the free fragment of the body of C-5 that has been displaced posteriorly into the vertebral canal. In addition to comminuted fractures of the body of C-5, there is also fracture of the lamina on the right side. Note the similarity between this case and Fig 5-26. *Source:* Reprinted with permission from ''The Posterior Vertebral Body Line: Importance in the Detection of Burst Fractures'' by RH Daffner, ZL Deeb, and WE Rothfus in *American Journal of Roentgenology* (1987;148:93–96), Copyright © 1987, American Roentgen Ray Society.

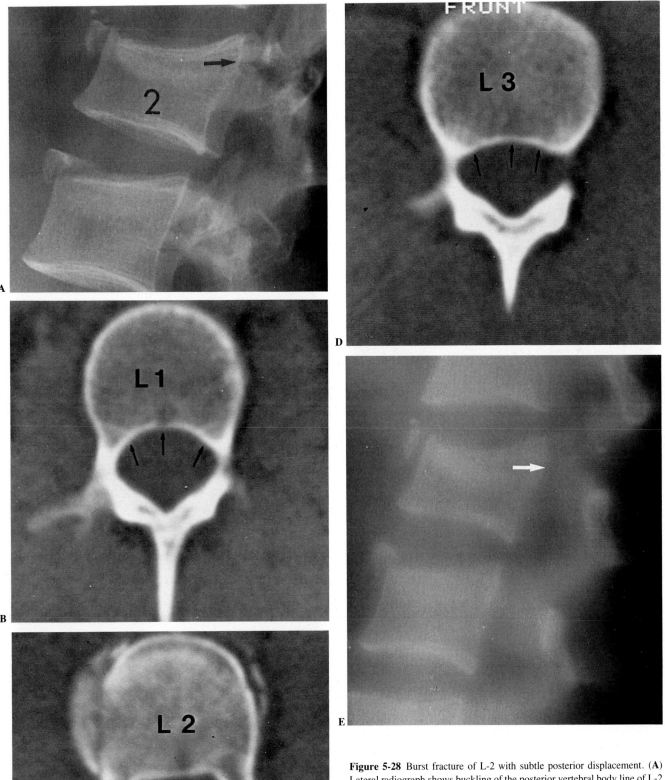

Figure 5-28 Burst fracture of L-2 with subtle posterior displacement. (**A**) Lateral radiograph shows buckling of the posterior vertebral body line of L-2 (arrow). In addition, there are fractures of the anterosuperior lips of the bodies of L2 and L-3. (**B**) CT scan through the inferior aspect of L-1 shows that the posterior vertebral line has a normal curvilinear shape (arrows). (**C**) CT section through the upper portion of the body of L-2 shows flattening of the posterior vertebral body (arrows), which accounts for the abnormality seen on the plain lateral radiograph. (**D**) CT section through L-3 shows the normal curvilinear appearance of the posterior vertebral body line. (**E**) Lateral tomogram shows the displaced fragment of L-2 (arrow).

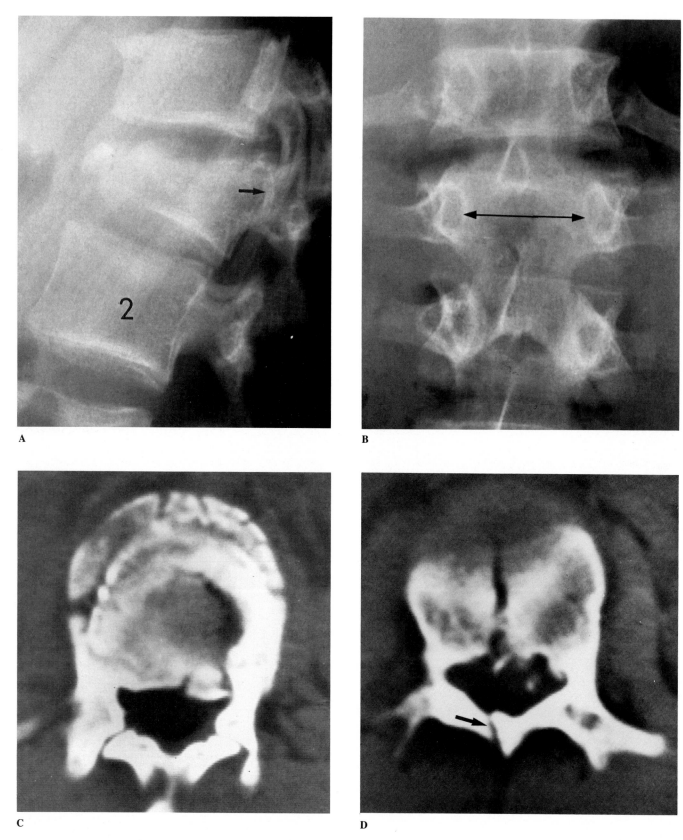

A

B

C

D

Figure 5-29 Burst fracture of L-1 with widening of the interpedicular distance. (**A**) Lateral radiograph shows compression and fragmentation of the body of L-1. The superior aspect of the posterior vertebral body line has been displaced posteriorly (arrow). (**B**) Frontal radiograph shows widening of the interpedicular distance of L-1 (double arrow). (**C**) CT scan through the upper portion of the vertebra shows a retropulsed fragment of the central portion of the body of L-1 encroaching on the vertebral canal. (**D**) CT scan through the lower portion of the vertebra shows vertical fracture through the body of L-1 combined with a fracture through the lamina of L-1 on the right (arrow). This accounts for the wide interpedicular distance. Note the multiple intracanalicular fragments.

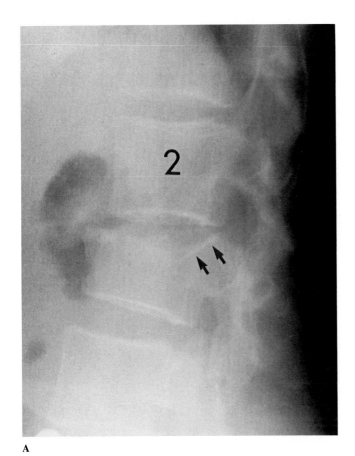

A

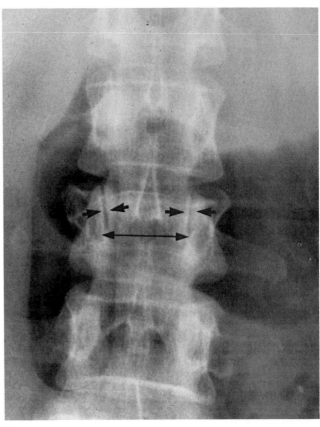

B

Figure 5-30 Burst fracture of L-3. (**A**) Lateral radiograph shows compression of the body of L-3 with fragmentation of the superior surface. There is rotation of a portion of the posterior vertebral body line (arrows). (**B**) Frontal radiograph shows widening of the interpedicular distance of L-3 (double arrow). There is also widening of the facet joints (short arrows).

Fractures of the upper sacrum occur quite commonly in conjunction with pelvic fractures. These fractures are frequently overlooked because of the superimposition of bowel gas and contents and because of the complex configuration of the sacrum. In 1982, Jackson and associates[16] described abnormalities of the arcuate lines of the sacrum that would indicate fractures. These archlike structures are easily visible on frontal radiographs of the pelvis and abdomen and represent the inferior surfaces of the bony struts that form the roofs of the anterior sacral foramina. Generally, the arcs of the first three segments are easily seen, but occasionally only the first two are visible (Fig 5-34). Fractures through the body of the sacrum result in disruption of these arcuate lines (Figs 5-35 and 5-36). Changes include frank disruption, angulation, or obliteration. A CT scan will confirm the presence of a fracture.[22]

Table 5-2 summarizes abnormalities of bony integrity.

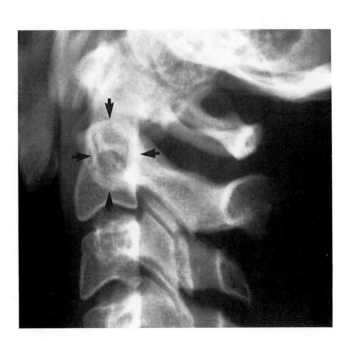

Figure 5-31 Normal lateral cervical radiograph showing ''Harris' ring'' (arrows).

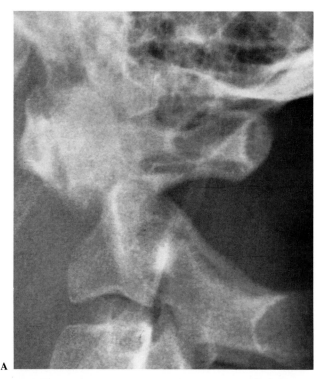

A

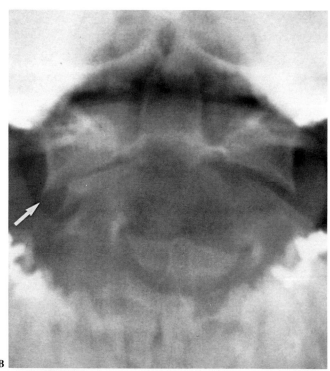

B

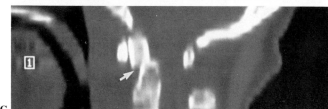

C

Figure 5-32 Dens fracture with anterior displacement. (**A**) Lateral radiograph shows a fracture at the base of the dens with anterior tilt and anterior displacement of the dens and C-1. Note the prevertebral soft tissue swelling. (**B**) Frontal radiograph shows that the base of the dens is indistinct. The superior portion of the dens appears to be larger because it is tilted and displaced anteriorly and is thus farther from the film on this AP radiograph. Note the lateral atlanto-axial offset on the right side (arrow). (**C**) CT reconstruction in the sagittal plane shows the displacement (arrow).

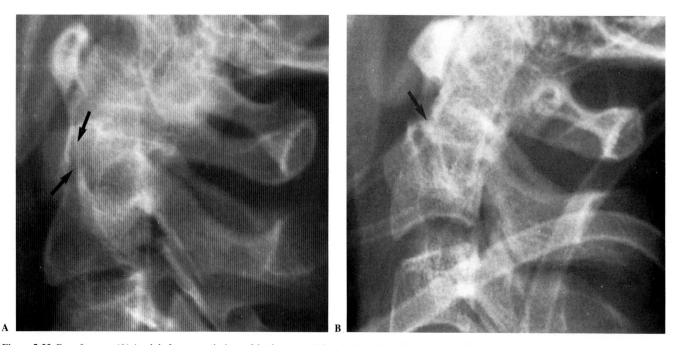

A   B

Figure 5-33 Dens fracture. (**A**) A subtle fracture at the base of the dens extends into the body. Note the disruption of ''Harris' ring'' (arrows). (**B**) In another patient with a similar injury, there is slight posterior displacement of the dens. Note the break in ''Harris' ring'' (arrow).

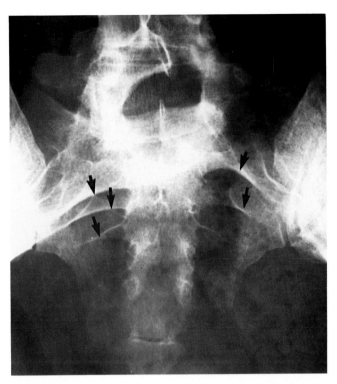

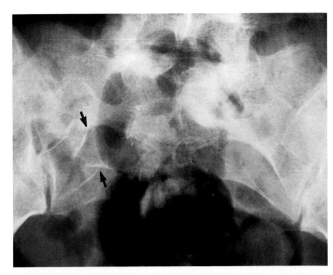

Figure 5-36 Right-sided sacral fractures manifesting as disruption of the sacral arcuate lines (arrows) in a patient with right-sided pelvic fractures.

Table 5-2 Abnormalities of Bony Integrity

Obvious fracture
Disruption of ring of C-2
"Fat" C-2 sign
Widening of interpedicular distance
Disruption of posterior vertebral body line
Disruption of sacral arcuate lines

Figure 5-34 Normal sacral arcuate lines (arrows) in a patient with congenital anomalies of L-5.

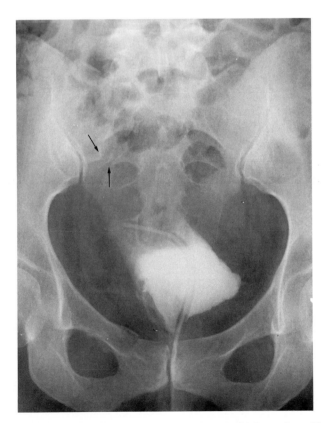

Figure 5-35 Subtle fracture of the sacrum on the right side in a patient with right-sided pelvic fractures. Note the disruption of the sacral arcuate lines (arrows). Compare with the opposite side.

CARTILAGE (JOINT) SPACE ABNORMALITIES

In general, injury to the vertebral column may produce an increase or a decrease in the width of the joint space. Increases in joint spaces are the most common. These changes include widening of the intervertebral disk space, widening of the interspinous distance, widening of the interpedicular distance, widening of the predental space, and widening of the facet joints. All these findings indicate severe ligamentous disruption. Joint spaces may also be narrowed. The most common manifestation of this occurs with flexion injuries, where the disk space above the compressed vertebra is narrowed (Fig 5-37). It must be remembered, however, that degenerative disease is the most common cause of disk space narrowing.

Widening of the intervertebral disk space, as mentioned in Chapter 4, is a common manifestation of extension injury (Figs 5-38 and 5-39).[6] This radiographic manifestation indicates damage to the anterior longitudinal ligament and to the disk itself.

Widening of the interspinous or interlaminar space is technically not a joint abnormality. Nevertheless, this finding typically accompanies severe flexion injuries and is associated with abnormalities in the facet joints themselves (Figs 5-40 and 5-41).[11,13,23,24] In addition to being visible on frontal and

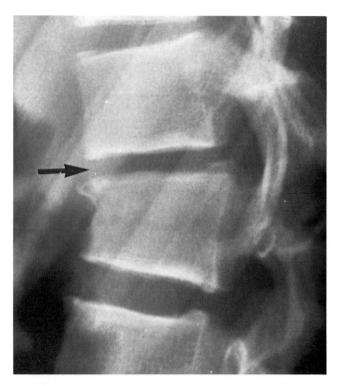

Figure 5-37 Compression fracture of L-1. In addition to flattening of the anterior aspect of the body of L-1, there is narrowing of the T-12 disk space (arrow).

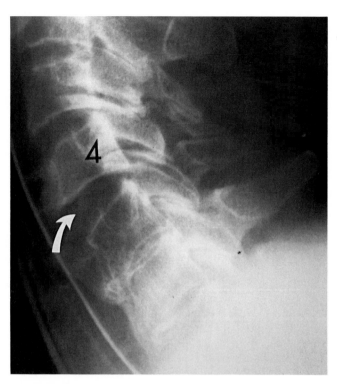

Figure 5-38 Extension injury at the C-4 disk level with widening of the C-4 disk space (arrow). The patient has diffuse idiopathic skeletal hyperostosis.

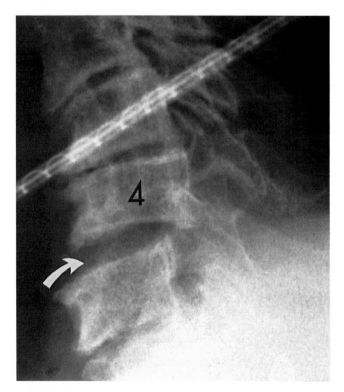

Figure 5-39 Extension injury in a patient with extensive degenerative change. There is widening of the C-4 disk space (curved arrow) along with retrolisthesis of C-4 on C-5.

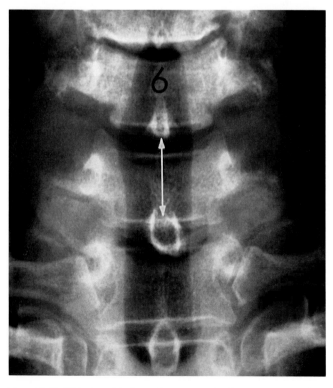

Figure 5-40 Widening of the interspinous space (double arrow) (same patient as in Fig 5-17).

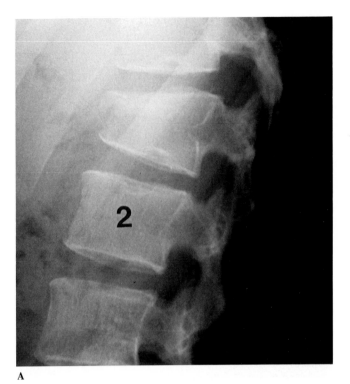

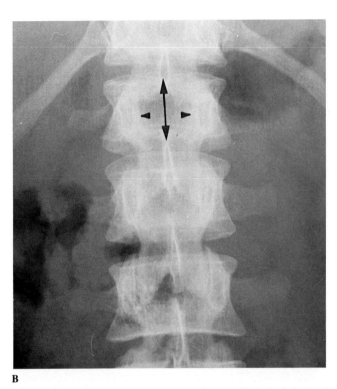

A   B

Figure 5-41 Burst fracture of L-1 with wide interspinous space. (**A**) Lateral radiograph shows compression of the anterior portion of the body of L-1. On the basis of the lateral radiograph alone, this appears to be a simple lumbar fracture. (**B**) Frontal radiograph shows widening of the interspinous space (double arrow). Note the naked facets of L-1 (arrowheads). These findings indicate that the patient has suffered a severe posterior ligamentous injury with resultant instability.

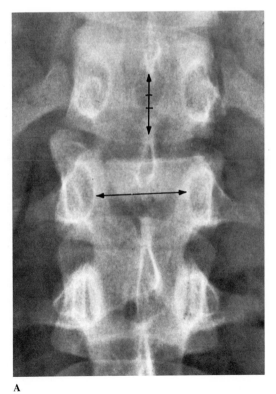

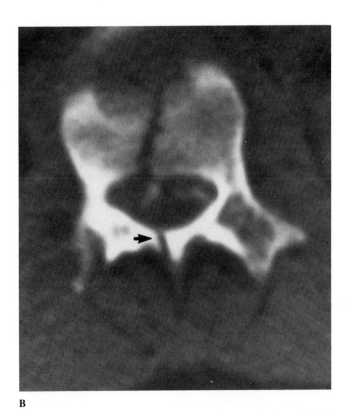

A   B

Figure 5-42 Burst fracture of L-1 with widening of the interpedicular space. (**A**) Frontal radiograph shows widening of the interpedicular space (horizontal double arrow). In addition, there is widening of the interspinous space between T-12 and L-1 (vertical double arrow). (**B**) CT scan shows a sagittal fracture through the body of L-1 as well as a fracture through the lamina on the left side (arrow).

lateral radiographs, it is manifest on CT scans by absence of the spinous process on two contiguous sections (Figs 5-40 and 5-41).

As mentioned earlier, the distance between the pedicles should not vary from one vertebral level to the next by more than 2 mm. This applies to both the transverse plane and the vertical plane. An increase in the transverse distance is an indication that the vertebra has been disrupted in the vertical plane with resultant bilateral lateral separation of the major fragments. This typically occurs in burst injuries (Figs 5-42 and 5-43). Widening of the interpedicular distance may be easily observed on frontal radiographs, and this finding usually accompanies widening of the facet joints of the involved vertebrae (Figs 5-42 and 5-43). The typical findings of a burst injury, including fragmentation, widened interspinous space, disrupted posterior vertebral body line, and narrowing of the superior disk space, are usually present. Disruption in the vertical plane indicates distraction or dislocation or both, usually from a flexion injury. Rotational and shearing injuries often produce similar changes.

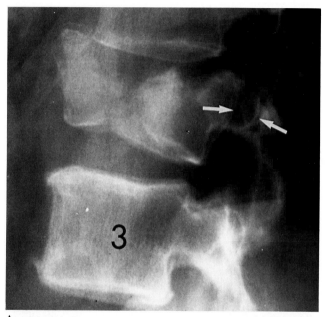

A

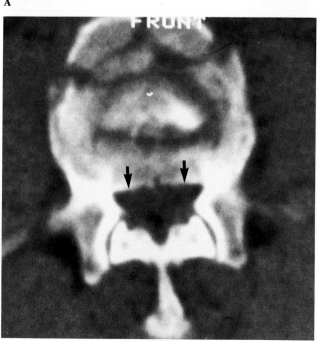

C

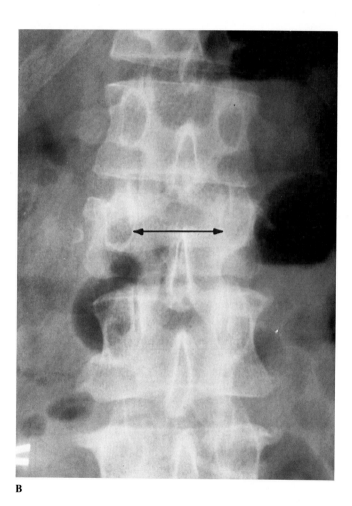

B

Figure 5-43 Burst fracture of L-2. (A) Lateral radiograph shows comminution of the body of L-2. There is retropulsion of bony fragments into the vertebral canal (arrows). (B) Frontal radiograph shows widening of the interpedicular distance (double arrow). (C) CT scan shows severe comminution of the body of L-1. There is retropulsion of bony fragments into the vertebral canal (arrows).

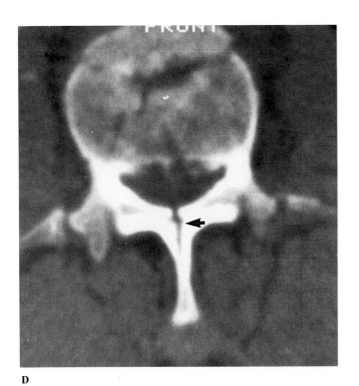

D

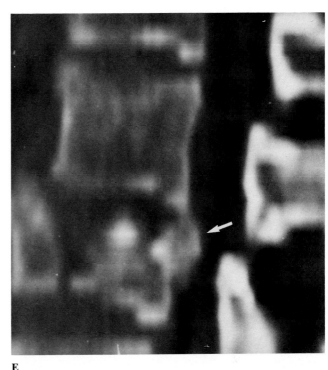

E

Figure 5-43 (**D**) CT scan at a lower level shows a vertical fracture through the lamina and spinous process (arrow). This allows the pedicles to widen. (**E**) Sagittal reconstruction shows the bony fragments within the vertebral canal (arrow).

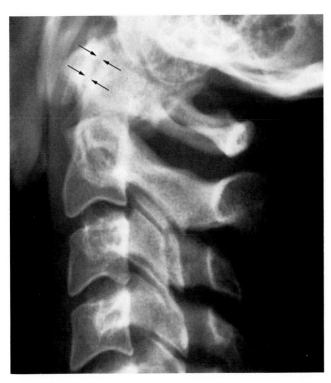

Figure 5-44 Normal predental space (arrows).

The predental space may be widened in injuries involving the check ligaments between C-1 and C-2. The predental space is measured from the anterior aspect of the dens to the posterior aspect of the anterior arch of the atlas. In adults, this measurement should never exceed 3 mm; in children it should not exceed 5 mm (Fig 5-44).[13,14,17,28] Widened predental space is most commonly encountered in patients with severe rheumatoid arthritis in whom synovial proliferation has resulted in destruction or disruption of the ligamentous attachments about the dens (Fig 5-45). True traumatic widening of this space is unusual (Fig 5-46).

The apophyseal or facet joints are often disrupted with severe flexion injuries.[13,24] In the typical case, there is forward luxation or dislocation of these facets (Fig 5-47). Complete disruption may result in unilateral (Fig 5-48) or bilateral (Fig 5-49) facet lock. Occasionally, the facet abnormality may be the only gross indication of an injury (Fig 5-50). In general, facet abnormalities occur in combination with other findings that indicate a flexion injury (Figs 5-37 to 5-43). "Naked" facets indicate severe ligamentous damage. This is often a manifestation of a severe flexion injury in the thoracolumbar region (Figs 5-51 and 5-52).

Table 5-3 summarizes cartilage or joint space abnormalities.

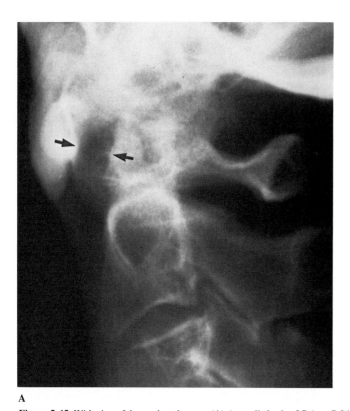

A

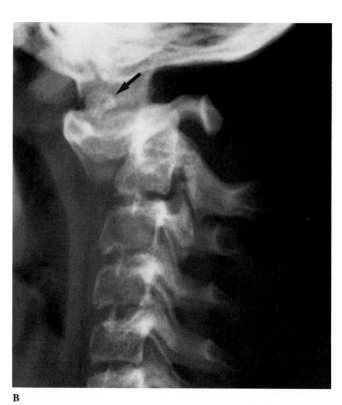

B

Figure 5-45 Widening of the predental space. (**A**) Anterolisthesis of C-1 on C-2 in a patient with rheumatoid arthritis. Note the wide predental space (arrows). (**B**) Wide predental space with dislocation of C-1 in a patient with os odontoideum (arrow).

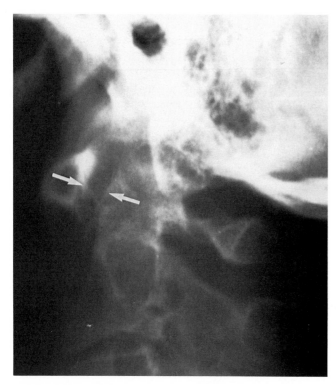

Figure 5-46 Posttraumatic widening of the predental space (arrows) in a patient with anterior luxation of C-1 on C-2.

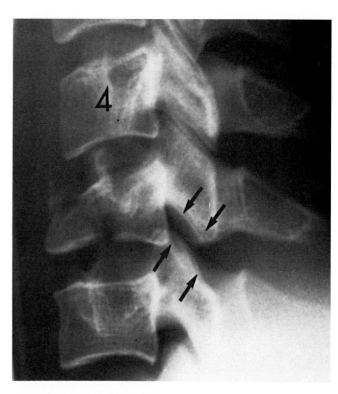

Figure 5-47 Widened facet joints (arrows) in a patient with a ''teardrop'' fracture of C-5 from a diving injury.

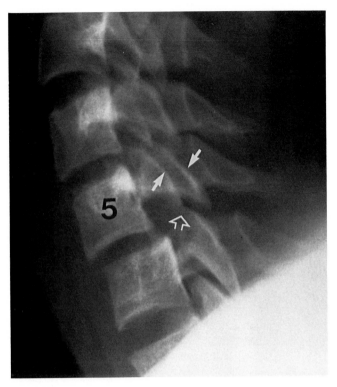

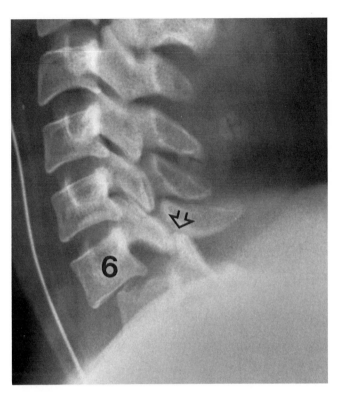

Figure 5-48 Unilateral facet lock at C5-6. Lateral radiograph shows slight anterolisthesis of C-5 on C-6. There is duplication of the facet images at C-5 (solid arrows) as well as at the levels above. The point of locking is indicated by the open arrow.

Figure 5-49 Anterior dislocation of C-6 on C-7 with bilateral facet locking (arrow).

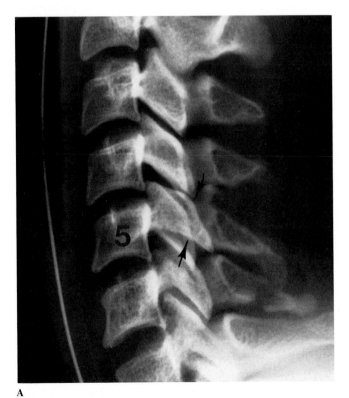

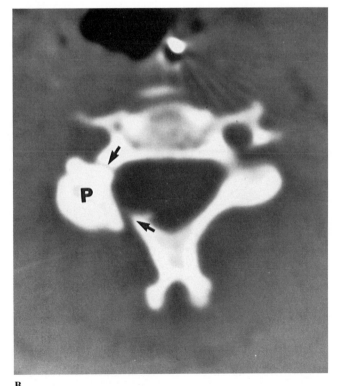

A

B

Figure 5-50 Lateral flexion injury with free-floating pillar of C-5. (**A**) Lateral radiograph shows duplication of the pillar image at C-5 (arrows). (**B**) CT scan shows fractures in the pedicle and lamina on the right side (arrows). The pillar (P) is rotated, resulting in an asymmetric image when compared to the left side.

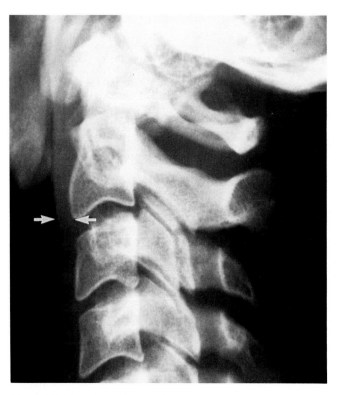

Figure 5-51 Normal retropharyngeal space.

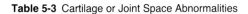

Table 5-3 Cartilage or Joint Space Abnormalities

Widening of predental space
Abnormal intervertebral disk space
Widening of apophyseal joints
"Naked" facets
Widening of interspinous or interlaminar distance
Abnormal Powers' ratio

SOFT TISSUE ABNORMALITIES

Injury to the vertebral column produces various soft tissue abnormalities. In many cases, these soft tissue findings may be the only indication of an occult fracture or subluxation. These findings include widening of the retropharyngeal space, widening of the retrotracheal space, displacement of the prevertebral fat stripe, soft tissue mass near the craniovertebral junction, deviation of the trachea or larynx, widening of the

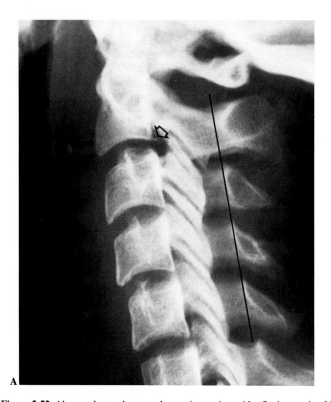

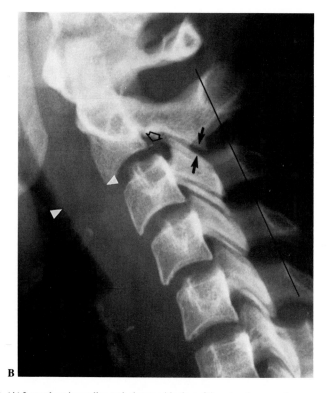

Figure 5-52 Abnormal retropharyngeal space in a patient with a flexion sprain of C2-3. (**A**) Lateral supine radiograph shows widening of the retropharyngeal space to 17 mm (double arrow). There is a small avulsion fracture off the posteroinferior base of the body of C-2 (open arrow). Note the malalignment of the spinolaminar line (drawn in). (**B**) Upright radiograph shows anterolisthesis of C-2 on C-3. There is widening of the facet joints of C2-3 (solid arrows). Note the small bony fragment from the posteroinferior lip of C-2 (open arrow) and the widening of the retropharyngeal space (arrowheads).

paraspinal soft tissue, and loss of the psoas stripe. The first five of these signs occur exclusively in the cervical region. Paraspinal soft tissue changes may be seen in the thoracic area, and loss of psoas stripe is observed within the lumbar region.[11,13]

The retropharyngeal space is measured from the anteroinferior aspect of the body of C-2 to the posterior aspect of the pharyngeal air column (Fig 5-51). This space should never exceed 7 mm in adults and children. In establishing this limit, magnification and technical factors are taken into account. Measurements are based on a lateral horizontal beam radiograph with a 40-in focal film distance. Disruptive injuries in this region produce widening of this space even in the absence of more obvious skeletal abnormalities (Figs 5-52 and 5-53).[11,13,31]

The retrotracheal space is measured from the anteroinferior aspect of the body of C-6 to the posterior tracheal wall (or shadow of the endotracheal tube (Figs 5-54 and 5-55). This space should never exceed 14 mm in children and 22 mm in adults. Again, measurements are based on standard 40-in radiographs made with the horizontal beam technique. As with widening of the retropharyngeal space, abnormality of the retrotracheal space accompanies severe disruptive injuries and may be the only clue to an occult injury (Figs 5-56 and 5-57).[11,13,31]

The prevertebral fat stripe courses caudally along the anterior surfaces of the vertebral bodies from C-2 through C-6 (Fig 5-57).[11,13,25,32] This thin band of fatty tissue parallels the anterior longitudinal ligament to the level of C-6, where it gradually deviates anteriorly and inferiorly toward the base of the neck. Displacement of this line from its normal location is a reliable indication that underlying injury has produced a hematoma (Figs 5-58 and 5-59).

Injury to the craniovertebral junction, C-1, or C-2 frequently produces a prevertebral hematoma that appears as a soft tissue mass anterior to C-1 and C-2 (Figs 5-60 and 5-61). This sign is a reliable indicator of injury when there is a history to support that diagnosis and a paucity of radiographic findings.[13]

Tracheal or laryngeal deviation is a nonspecific sign and may occur under various circumstances besides trauma. These airway structures are not securely fixed in the neck and are subject to motion not only by posttraumatic hematoma but also by infection. This sign should not be relied on solely as a basis for a diagnosis of injury (Fig 5-62).

Paraspinal soft tissue changes are an indication that an occult injury may have occurred in the thoracic region. This is particularly true in obese individuals with high thoracic fractures (Fig 5-63). This sign is by no means specific for injury

(text continues on p. 132)

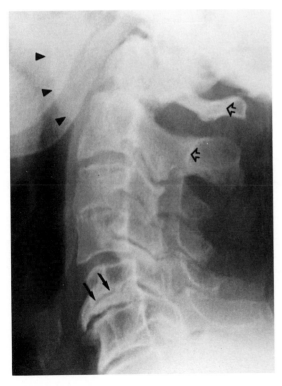

Figure 5-53 Prevertebral hematoma at C1-2 (arrowheads). This patient has a fracture of the dens with retrolisthesis of the dens and C-1 on C-2. Note the malalignment of the spinolaminar line (open arrows). The oblique lucency over the body of C-5 (solid arrows) is a Mach band due to osteophytes along the vertebral margin (see Chapter 6 for description).

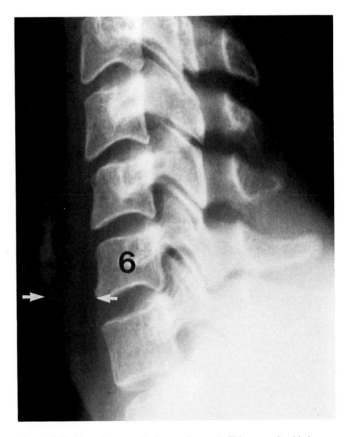

Figure 5-54 Normal retrotracheal space (arrows). This space should always be less than two-thirds of the width of the body of C-6.

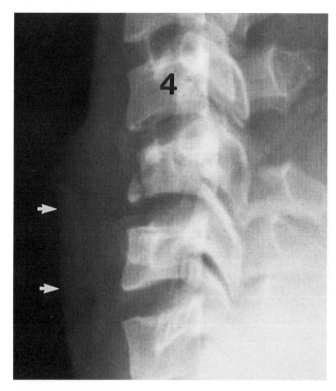

Figure 5-55 Retrotracheal hemorrhage with widening of the retrotracheal space in a patient with a burst fracture of C-5. Note the retrotracheal hematoma (arrows).

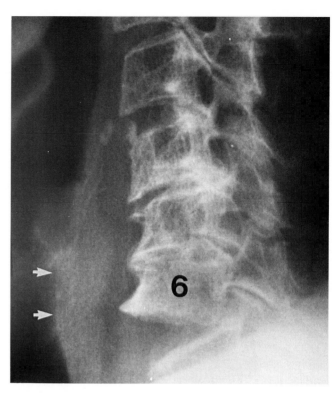

Figure 5-56 Retrotracheal hemorrhage in a patient with extension injury of C6-7. Note the retrotracheal hematoma (arrows). There is also widening of the C-6 disk space.

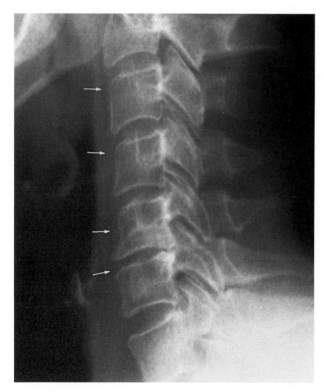

Figure 5-57 Normal prevertebral fat stripe (arrows).

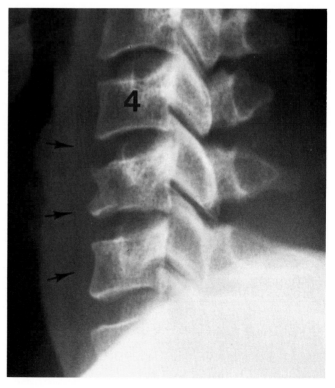

Figure 5-58 Displacement of the prevertebral fat stripe (arrows) by prevertebral hematoma resulting from a compression fracture of C-5.

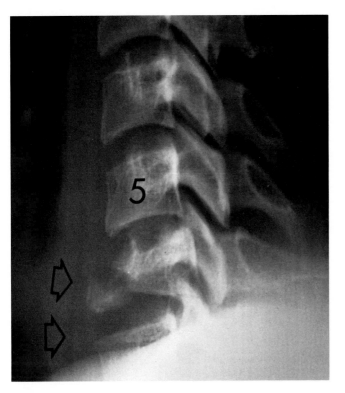

Figure 5-59 Displaced prevertebral fat stripe (arrows) in a patient with a burst fracture of C-6.

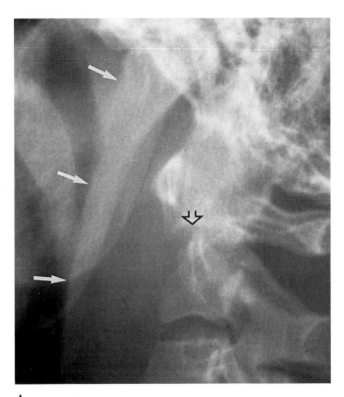

A

Figure 5-60 Dens fracture. (**A**) Lateral radiograph shows prevertebral hematoma (solid arrows). There is a dens fracture (open arrow) with slight anterior displacement.

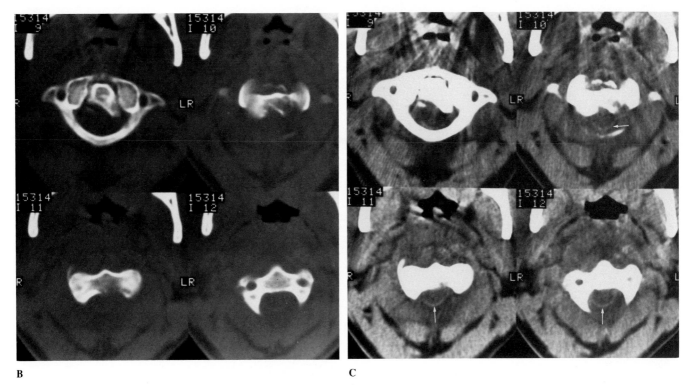

B

C

Figure 5-60 (**B**) CT scan at bone windows shows the fracture at the base of the dens and the prevertebral hematoma. (**C**) Soft tissue windows show subarachnoid blood (arrows).

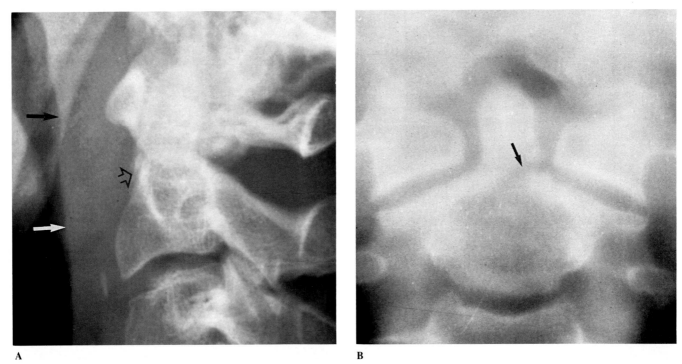

A   B

Figure 5-61 Dens fracture with prevertebral hematoma. (**A**) Lateral radiograph shows soft tissue swelling anteriorly (solid arrows). The dens fracture (open arrow) is subtle. (**B**) Frontal tomogram shows the fracture (arrow).

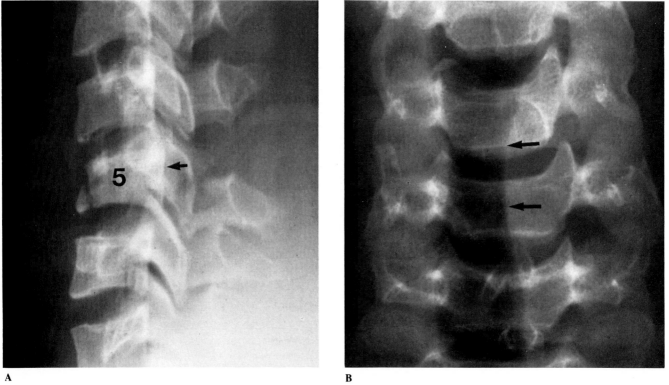

A   B

Figure 5-62 Tracheal deviation in a patient with a burst fracture. (**A**) Lateral radiograph shows a burst fracture of C-5. A fragment of bone has been displaced posteriorly (arrow). (**B**) Frontal radiograph shows tracheal deviation (arrows) as a result of the prevertebral hematoma.

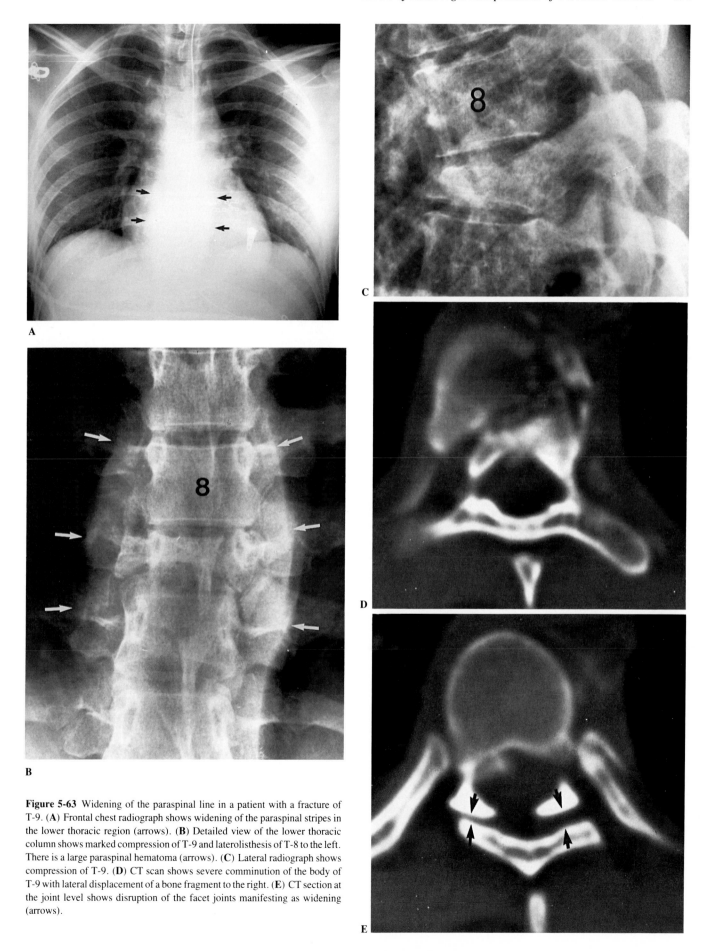

Figure 5-63 Widening of the paraspinal line in a patient with a fracture of T-9. (**A**) Frontal chest radiograph shows widening of the paraspinal stripes in the lower thoracic region (arrows). (**B**) Detailed view of the lower thoracic column shows marked compression of T-9 and laterolisthesis of T-8 to the left. There is a large paraspinal hematoma (arrows). (**C**) Lateral radiograph shows compression of T-9. (**D**) CT scan shows severe comminution of the body of T-9 with lateral displacement of a bone fragment to the right. (**E**) CT section at the joint level shows disruption of the facet joints manifesting as widening (arrows).

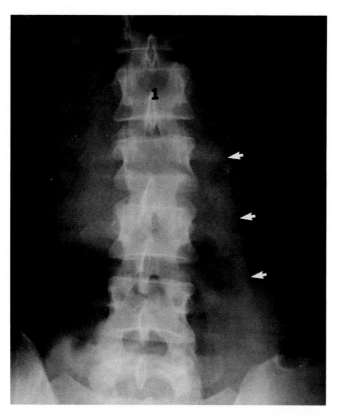

Figure 5-64 Loss of psoas stripe in a patient who suffered a seatbelt-type injury of L-2. Frontal radiograph shows the normal psoas stripe on the left (arrows). This stripe has been obliterated on the right.

and also occurs in infections, neoplasms, or extramedullary hematopoiesis.

Loss of the psoas stripe is another nonspecific finding that may occasionally be useful in diagnosing an occult lumbar injury. Generally there is some other indication that injury has occurred (Fig 5-64). This sign may also occur with infections or spasm of any etiology.

Table 5-4 summarizes soft tissue abnormalities.

THE "RULES OF 2s"

Throughout this and the preceding chapters, a number of measurements have been given in which 2 mm is the maximum distance allowable for that particular diagnostic parameter. These may be summarized as the "rules of 2s." This distance has been determined from observation of thousands of radiographs with technical parameters as well as clinical findings taken into consideration. Although exceptions may be found, the 2-mm rule remains valid in most cases.

Two millimeters is the maximum allowable difference between the interspinous or interlaminar spaces of three contiguous levels. Two millimeters is the maximum allowable

Table 5-4 Soft Tissue Abnormalities

Widening of retropharyngeal space
Widening of retrotracheal space
Displacement of prevertebral fat stripe
Soft tissue mass in craniocervical junction
Deviation of trachea or laryngx
Paraspinal soft tissue mass
Loss of psoas stripe

difference in the interpedicular distance between two contiguous levels. This applies not only to the transverse interpedicular distance but also to the vertical interpedicular distance.

In the atlanto-axial region, 2 mm is the maximum allowable unilateral or bilateral lateral atlanto-axial offset between the lateral masses of C-1 and the body of C-2 on the frontal view. This is most likely to occur in the presence of some form of arch anomaly of C-1.[12] Jefferson fractures, as previously mentioned, produce offset of 3 mm or more.

Lateral flexion and extension views, particularly in the cervical region, may produce up to 2 mm of anterolisthesis or retrolisthesis. This is due to simple ligamentous laxity of the anterior or posterior longitudinal ligaments and is believed to be of no clinical significance as long as the spinolaminar line remains intact.

The normal facet joints should never exceed 2 mm in width, particularly in flexion. Any increase is usually the result of a posterior ligamentous disruption.

Finally, there are normal differences in the heights of the anterior portions and posterior portions of the thoracic and lumbar vertebral bodies. The anterior margins of thoracic vertebral bodies are 2 mm shorter than the posterior margins. This accounts for the thoracic kyphosis. Conversely, the posterior portions of the lumbar vertebral bodies are up to 2 mm shorter than the anterior portions; this accounts for the lumbar lordosis.

Table 5-5 summarizes the "rules of 2s."

Table 5-5 "Rules of 2s"

Two millimeters is the normal upper limit of difference for:

1. interspinous or interlaminar space
2. interpedicular distance (transverse and vertical)
3. unilateral or bilateral lateral atlanto-axial offset
4. anterolisthesis or retrolisthesis with flexion or extension
5. facet joint width
6. height of anterior and posterior thoracic and lumbar vertebral bodies

REFERENCES

1. Amyes EW, Anderson FM: Fracture of the odontoid process: Report of sixty-three cases. *Arch Surg* 1956;72:377–393.

2. Anderson LD, D'Alonzo RT: Fractures of the odontoid process of the axis. *J Bone Joint Surg* 1974;56A:1663–1674.

3. Atlas SW, Regenbogen V, Rogers LF, et al: The radiographic characterization of burst fractures of the spine. *AJR* 1986;147:575–582.

4. Braakman R, Vinken PJ: Unilateral facet interlocking in the lower cervical spine. *J Bone Joint Surg* 1967;49B:249–257.

5. Cattell HS, Filtzer DL: Pseudosubluxation and other normal variations of the cervical spine in children: A study of one hundred and sixty children. *J Bone Joint Surg* 1965;47A:1295–1309.

6. Cintron E, Gilula LA, Murphy WA, et al: The widened disk space: A sign of cervical hyperextension injury. *Radiology* 1981;141:639–644.

7. Clark WM, Gehweiler JA Jr, Laib R: Twelve significant signs of cervical spine trauma. *Skeletal Radiol* 1979;3:201–205.

8. Daffner RH, Deeb ZL, Rothfus WE: "Fingerprints" of vertebral trauma—A unifying concept based on mechanisms. *Skeletal Radiol* 1986;15:518–525.

9. Daffner RH, Deeb ZL, Rothfus WE: The posterior vertebral body line: Importance in the detection of burst fractures. *AJR* 1987;148:93–96.

10. Dolan KD: Cervicobasilar relationships. *Radiol Clin North Am* 1977;15:155–166.

11. Gehweiler JA Jr, Daffner RH, Osborne RL Jr: Relevant signs of stable and unstable thoracolumbar vertebral column trauma. *Skeletal Radiol* 1981;7:179–183.

12. Gehweiler JA Jr, Daffner RH, Roberts L Jr: Malformations of the atlas vertebra simulating the Jefferson fracture. *AJR* 1983;140:1083–1086.

13. Gehweiler JA Jr, Osborne RL Jr, Becker RF: *The Radiology of Vertebral Trauma*. Philadelphia, WB Saunders, 1980.

14. Greenberg AD: Atlantoaxial dislocations. *Brain* 1968;91:665–684.

15. Harris JH Jr, Burke JT, Ray RD, et al: Low (type III) odontoid fracture: A new radiographic sign. *Radiology* 1984;153:353–356.

16. Jackson H, Kam J, Harris JH Jr, et al: The sacral arcuate lines in upper sacral fractures. *Radiology* 1982;145:35–39.

17. Jacobson G, Alder DC: An evaluation of lateral atlanto-axial displacement in injuries of the cervical spine. *Radiology* 1953;61:355–362.

18. Jacobson G, Bleecker HH: Pseudosubluxation of the axis in children. *AJR* 1959;82:472–481.

19. Jefferson G: Fracture of the atlas vertebra: Report of four cases, and a review of those previously recorded. *Br J Surg* 1920;7:407–422.

20. Lee C, Woodring JH, Goldstein SJ, et al: Evaluation of traumatic atlantooccipital dislocations. *AJNR* 1987;8:19–26.

21. Lee C, Woodring JH, Rogers LF, et al: The radiographic distinction of degenerative slippage (spondylolisthesis and retrolisthesis) from traumatic slippage of the cervical spine. *Skeletal Radiol* 1986;15:439–443.

22. Montana MA, Richardson ML, Kilcoyne RF, et al: CT of sacral injury. *Radiology* 1986;161:499–503.

23. Naidich JB, Naidich TP, Garfein C, et al: The widened interspinous distance: A useful sign of anterior cervical dislocation in the supine frontal projection. *Radiology* 1977;123:113–116.

24. O'Callaghan JP, Ullrich CG, Yuan HA, et al: CT of facet distraction in flexion injuries of the thoracolumbar spine: The "naked" facet. *AJNR* 1980;1:97–102.

25. Penning L: Prevertebral hematoma in cervical spine injury: Incidence and etiologic significance. *AJR* 1981;136:553–561.

26. Powers B, Miller MD, Kramer RS, et al: Traumatic anterior atlanto-occipital dislocation. *Neurosurgery* 1979;4:12–17.

27. Schaaf RE, Gehweiler JA Jr, Powers B, et al: Lateral hyperflexion injuries of the spine. *Skeletal Radiol* 1978;3:73–78.

28. Shapiro R, Youngberg AS, Rothman SL: The differential diagnosis of traumatic lesions of the occipito-atlanto-axial segment. *Radiol Clin North Am* 1973;11:505–526.

29. Smoker WRK, Dolan KD: The "fat" C2: A sign of fracture. *AJNR* 1987;8:33–38.

30. Suss RA, Zimmerman RD, Leeds NE: Pseudospread of the atlas: False sign of Jefferson fracture in young children. *AJNR* 1983;4:183–186.

31. Templeton PA, Young JWR, Mirvis SE, et al: The value of retropharyngeal soft tissue measurements in trauma of the adult cervical spine. *Skeletal Radiol* 1987;16:98–104.

32. Whalen JP, Woodruff CL: The cervical prevertebral fat stripe: A new aid in evaluating the cervical prevertebral soft tissue space. *AJR* 1970;109:445–451.

Chapter 6

Pseudofractures and
Normal Variants

The preceding chapters discussed the diagnosis of fractures of the vertebral column. This chapter explores entities that are often confused with fractures and may, in fact, be misdiagnosed as fractures. It is just as important for the radiologist and referring physician to be familiar with pseudofractures and normal variants that may simulate fractures as it is for them to be able to recognize fractures.[11,13]

PSEUDOFRACTURES

Pseudofractures are among a group of illusory phenomena that result from overlapping images, differences in background illumination, subjective contour formation, and parallax effect.[1] The value of the interpretation of any imaging study is determined by the ability of the observer to assess correctly the shadows contributing to the image on the film. Furthermore, the makeup of that image represents a composite of the shadows of all the structures contained within the plane of that image. Illusory phenomena result in various false images that are often interpreted as resulting from some significant pathologic abnormality. With the exception of the parallax effect, which results from the location of real structures in relation to the x-ray beam, all the other phenomena are due to the Mach effect.[1-3,5]

Image perception is a complex process that depends on input from optical, anatomical, physiological, and psychological factors. Basic optical factors include the size of the object and its contour, the type of illumination (direct or background), color, and adjacent shading. Anatomical factors include the information-gathering structures (cornea, iris, and lens), the reception system (rods and cones of the retina), and the processing system (optic nerve, optic tract, and visual cortex). The physiological components include the sensitivity of the rods and cones to stimulation and effect of lateral inhibition. The psychological factors are those that make it possible to interpret visual data and are based on previous learning experiences. The final component of image interpretation is that of perceptual learning. The novice to radiologic interpretation sees the same images on a radiograph that an experienced radiologist sees. The learning process, however, teaches the culling out of important information from the irrelevant and the collation of findings on the study with a pathologic process that will account for those changes.[1]

Mach Bands

Mach bands are a perceptual phenomenon in which bright and dark "lines" appear at the borders of structures of different optical (radiographic) density. Because they are observed

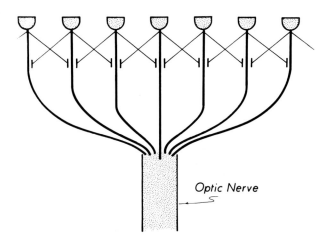

Figure 6-1 Schematic drawing of the neural pathways through the retina. The heavy lines represent the primary afferent neurons to the optic nerve. The small lines represent an interlacing network of fibers that carry inhibitory impulses to each of the neighboring primary neurons. Impulses passing along these fibers result in lateral inhibition. *Source*: Reprinted with permission from "Visual Illusions Affecting Perception of the Roentgen Image" by RH Daffner in *CRC Critical Reviews in Diagnostic Imaging* (1983;20:79–119), Copyright © 1983, CRC Press Inc, Boca Raton, FL.

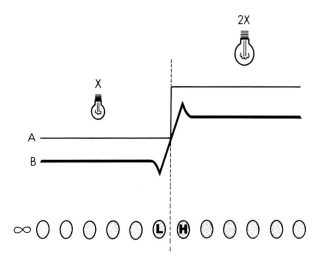

Figure 6-3 Mach band formation. *Source*: Reprinted with permission from "Pseudofracture of the Dens: Mach Bands" by RH Daffner in *American Journal of Roentgenology* (1977;128:607–612), Copyright © 1977, American Roentgen Ray Society.

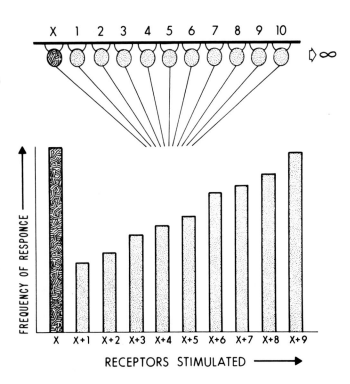

Figure 6-2 Effect of lateral inhibition. *Source*: Reprinted with permission from "Visual Illusions Affecting Perception of the Roentgen Image" by RH Daffner in *CRC Critical Reviews in Diagnostic Imaging* (1983;20:79–119). Copyright © 1983, CRC Press Inc, Boca Raton, FL.

in any situation where a half-shadow or penumbra is cast, they are found in radiological studies along the borders of structures of different radiodensity.

Ernst Mach (1838-1916) was an Austrian physicist-philosopher-psychologist who accidently discovered the phenomenon bearing his name in 1865. His original formulation predated by nearly a century the discovery of the neural inhibitory interactions within the retina and other portions of the nervous system whence the phenomena originate.[1,2]

Mach bands occur as the result of the process of lateral inhibition. A histologic section through the retina reveals an intricate meshwork of nerve fibers. In addition to the primary afferent neurons from each receptor, there is a fine network of fibers from the primary neuron to its neighbors (Fig 6-1). Impulses passing along these fibers result in an inhibitory effect on the neighboring primary neurons. The effect of this inhibitory response is illustrated in Fig 6-2. If receptor X is stimulated and its response alone is recorded, that response is as shown on the shaded portion of Fig 6-2. If receptor X and receptor 1 are both stimulated and the response from receptor X alone is recorded, that response is for X + 1. Similarly, stimulating receptor X and any of the other receptors and recording the response from receptor X produces a gradation of responses. Figure 6-2 illustrates two points: the closer two receptors are, the greater the inhibitory effect; and the greater the separation between receptors, the less powerful the inhibitory effect.[1,2]

The actual formation of negative (dark) and positive (light) Mach bands is illustrated in Fig 6-3. In this illustration, two sets of light receptors separated by a barrier are exposed to low-intensity (X) and high-intensity (2X) light sources.

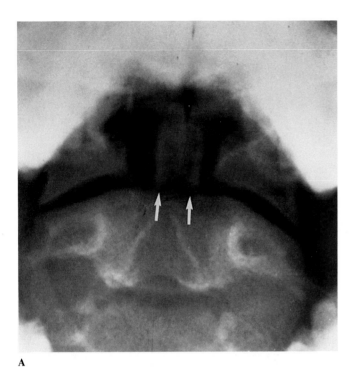
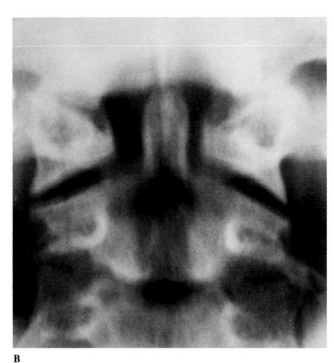

A   B

Figure 6-4 Mach band at the base of dens. **(A)** This pseudofracture (arrows) is the most common of all encountered in skeletal radiology. In this instance, the abnormality is caused by the overlap of the shadow of the anterior arch of the atlas. The lateral radiograph was normal. **(B)** Tomogram through the dens shows no evidence of fracture. *Source:* Reprinted with permission from ''Pseudofracture of the Dens: Mach Bands'' by RH Daffner in *American Journal of Roentgenology* (1977;128:607–612), Copyright © 1977, American Roentgen Ray Society.

Because of the barrier, no overlap occurs between those receptors receiving low-intensity stimulation and those receiving high-intensity stimulation. Line A is the response curve that would be recorded if lateral inhibition did not occur. Note that the response to those receptors receiving higher stimulation is higher. Because of lateral inhibition, however, the actual response curve is that shown in B. The difference in expected response and actual response is greater on the side receiving the greater stimulation. This is due to the fact that the greater the amount of stimulation, the greater the degree of lateral inhibition. Conversely, the less intense the stimulation, the less pronounced the degree of inhibition.

Adjacent to the midline there is a dip in response for receptor L, which was receiving low stimulation, and a peak in responses for receptor H, which received high stimulation. A mathematical model can designate the degree of inhibition for each receptor on the low side as $i + i = 2i$; for the receptors receiving high stimulation, the amount of inhibition is $2i + 2i = 4i$. The border receptors (L and H) are also inhibited by fibers from their neighbors. Receptor L receives inhibitory impulses not only from its neighbors but also from receptor H. Thus the total inhibitory effect on receptor L is $i + 2i = 3i$. Since the recorded response from receptor L is less than that of its neighbors, a dip is recorded in the curve, and this appears as a negative or dark Mach band. Conversely, on the high-

intensity side receptor H is inhibited by its neighbors as well as by receptor L. The total inhibitory effect here is also $3i$. Since this is less than the total inhibitory effect on the other receptors on that side, however, the recorded response is greater and appears as a spike or a positive or light Mach band.[1,2]

Clinical Applications of Mach Bands

Most radiologists are familiar with the contrast-enhancing effect Mach bands have in various areas of the body. As mentioned above, the formation of Mach bands is favored in any situation where there is overlap of shadows of structures of different radiodensity. Mach bands actually aid in the interpretation of radiographs in most instances by providing apparent enhanced borders of structures. In the skeleton, however, Mach bands may cause considerable diagnostic difficulty. Most of these skeletal aberrations are found in the vertebral column.[1–3,5,9]

The best known skeletal Mach band occurs at the base of the dens, where a thin lucent line may be misinterpreted as a fracture (Figs 6-4 to 6-6). The overlapping structures that are most likely to produce this phenomenon are the posterior arch of the atlas, the occiput, skin folds in the neck, and, occasionally, air over the back of the tongue.[1,2] The lateral radiograph

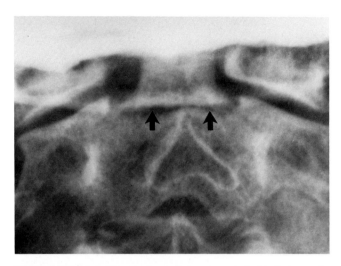

Figure 6-5 Mach band at the base of dens (arrow). In this instance, the lucency was caused by the overlap of the arch of the atlas. The lucency is continuous with the shadow of that structure.

of the same region is most useful for resolving the problem because, in the presence of a Mach band on the frontal view, there is no evidence of fracture on the lateral view, Harris' ring is intact, the body of C-2 is not "fat," and there are no abnormal soft tissue changes in the predental region (Figs 6-4 to 6-6). In many instances the Mach band may be traced to the shadow of the arch of the atlas, which extends laterally beyond the dens (Fig 6-5). In some instances when doubt remains as to the veracity of the lucency, tomography may be necessary (Fig 6-6).

True fractures of the dens usually show anterior or posterior displacement (Figs 6-7 and 6-8). In almost every instance of a dens fracture, there is disruption of Harris' ring and soft tissue swelling in the predental region (Figs 6-7 to 6-9). Furthermore, a fracture is usually easily visible in both the frontal and lateral views. Tomograms, if necessary, clearly delineate the abnormality.

Overlapping shadows of the incisor teeth may produce another Mach band of the dens (Fig 6-10). This abnormality is not difficult to diagnose when the interfering shadows are traced. The lateral radiograph is normal.

On an oblique view of the cervical column, overlapping shadows of the posterior arches of the vertebrae may result in Mach band formation (Fig 6-11). This may be observed at any level. A lateral radiograph, or occasionally a CT scan, may be necessary to resolve this situation.

Lower in the cervical column, the shadows of the uncinate processes abutting the undersurface of the vertebral bodies may result in a spurious lucency appearing on the lateral radiograph (Fig 6-12). This lucency is probably the second most common Mach band encountered in the vertebral column and is constant in its location.[3,5] It should not be confused with

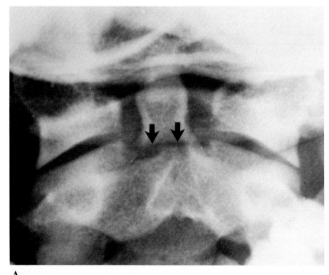

A

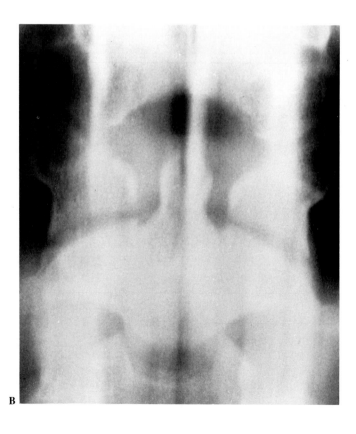

B

Figure 6-6 Mach band at C-2. **(A)** Frontal radiograph shows a lucency across the base of the dens (arrows). This is in continuity with the shadow of the arch of the atlas. The lucency below the arrow on the right, due to air trapped within the folds of the tongue, caused additional diagnostic difficulty. The lateral radiograph was normal. **(B)** Tomogram through the dens shows no evidence of fracture. *Source:* Reprinted with permission from "Pseudofracture of the Dens: Mach Bands" by RH Daffner in *American Journal of Roentgenology* (1977;128:607–612), Copyright © 1977, American Roentgen Ray Society.

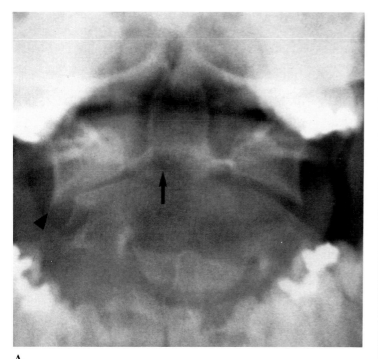
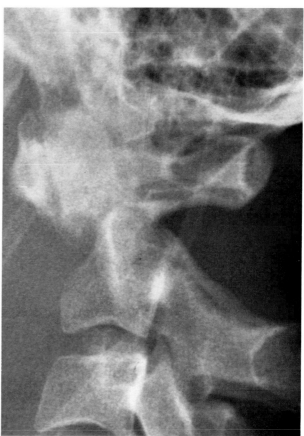

A

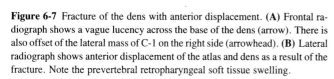

Figure 6-7 Fracture of the dens with anterior displacement. (**A**) Frontal radiograph shows a vague lucency across the base of the dens (arrow). There is also offset of the lateral mass of C-1 on the right side (arrowhead). (**B**) Lateral radiograph shows anterior displacement of the atlas and dens as a result of the fracture. Note the prevertebral retropharyngeal soft tissue swelling.

B

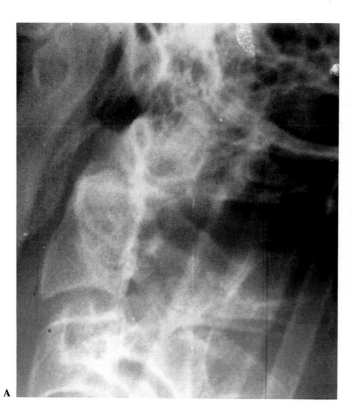
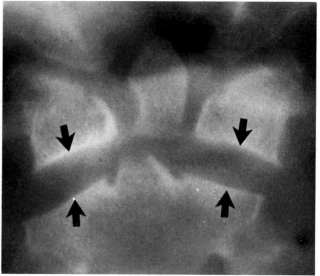

B

Figure 6-8 Dens fracture with posterior displacement. (**A**) Lateral radiograph shows that the dens is sheared off at its base with posterior displacement. (**B**) Frontal tomogram shows the displacement as well as marked widening of the joint space between the lateral masses of C-1 and the body of C-2 (arrows).

A

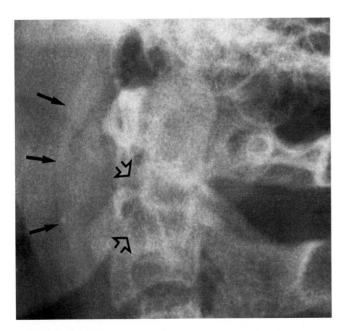

Figure 6-9 Subtle dens fracture. The main manifestation of this fracture is the disruption of ''Harris' ring'' (open arrows). Note the prevertebral soft tissue swelling (solid arrows). The lateral film is invaluable in determining whether a dens fracture or a Mach band is present.

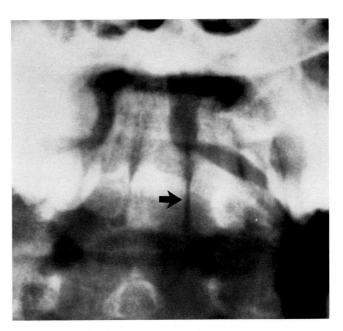

Figure 6-10 Mach band due to tooth margins. There is a vertical lucency across the left side of the body of C-2 (arrow) due to the margins of two incisor teeth. This is a common radiographic finding in patients in whom the atlanto-axial view is not properly positioned.

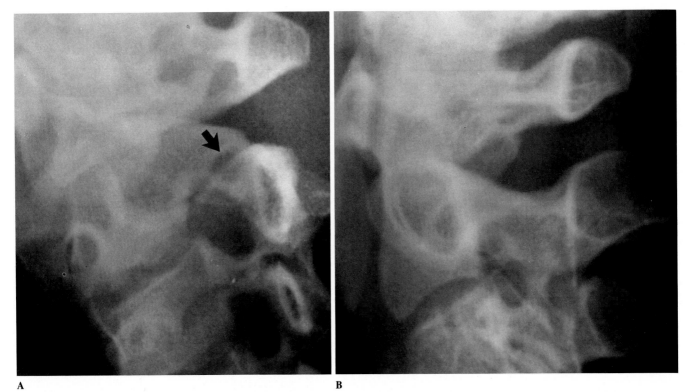

A   B

Figure 6-11 Mach band of the posterior arch of C-2. **(A)** The trauma oblique radiograph shows a lucency across the posterior arch of C-2 on the left (arrow). This is due to the overlapping shadows of the arches of the axis in this position. **(B)** A lateral radiograph shows no evidence of fracture in the lamina of C-2.

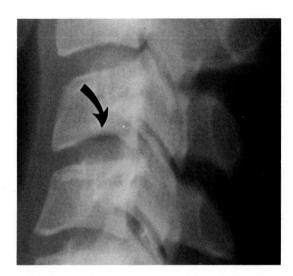

Figure 6-12 Mach band due to the proximity of the uncinate process and the vertebral body above. There is a horizontal lucency beneath the body of C-3 (arrow). There is no prevertebral soft tissue swelling to indicate injury. This is a common normal finding on lateral cervical radiographs. *Source*: Reprinted with permission from ''Pseudovacuum of the Cervical Intervertebral Disc: A Normal Variant'' by RH Daffner and JA Gehweiler Jr in *American Journal of Roentgenology* (1981;137:737–739), Copyright © 1981, American Roentgen Ray Society.

the less common disk bond injury (Fig 6-13), which results in a lucency adjacent to the lower anterior aspect of the intervertebral disk space.

Prominent transverse processes whose shadows overlap the vertebral bodies may result in Mach band formation on the lateral radiograph in the cervical vertebral column (Fig 6-14). Similarly, spurs from uncinate processes (Fig 6-15) or large osteophytes projecting off the lateral margins of the vertebral bodies (Fig 6-16) may produce pseudofractures running horizontally or obliquely across the mid to posterior portion of vertebral bodies.[5,9] These findings, too, are extremely common, particularly in elderly individuals. Once again, it may be necessary to resort to lateral tomography to resolve such a situation.

The overlap of air within the recesses of the larynx may, on occasion, be misinterpreted as a fracture of a cervical vertebra. This is not a Mach band. A curious pseudofracture produced by overlapping shadows of the sternum on the thoracic vertebral column (Fig 6-17) is a true Mach band. By carefully following the contour of the lucency, it is possible to see that it continues with the sternum. As always, in difficult cases it may be necessary to employ conventional tomography or CT to resolve the situation.

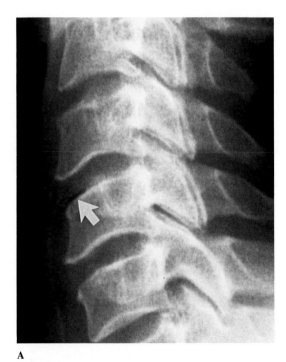

A

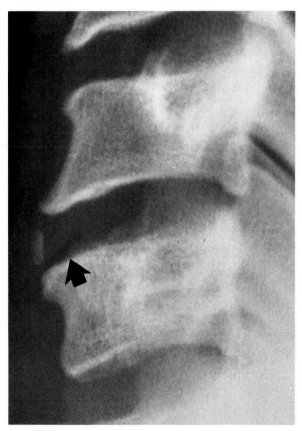

B

Figure 6-13 Disk bond injuries. Compare these cases with that in Fig 6-12. **(A)** There is a linear lucency just above the anterosuperior aspect of the body of C-5 (arrow). This is a true disk bond injury due to extension. **(B)** A similar finding in another patient (arrow).

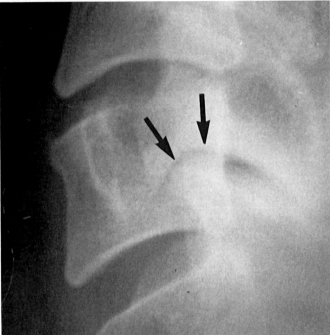

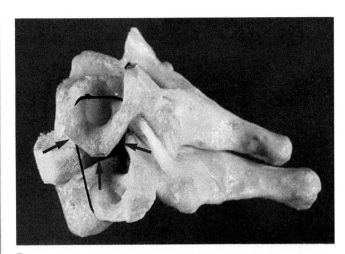

B

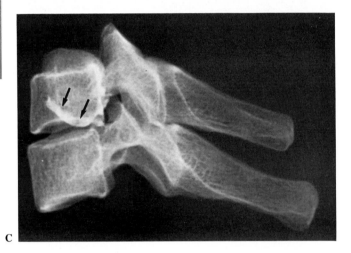

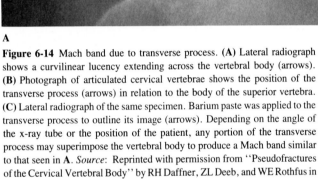

A

Figure 6-14 Mach band due to transverse process. **(A)** Lateral radiograph shows a curvilinear lucency extending across the vertebral body (arrows). **(B)** Photograph of articulated cervical vertebrae shows the position of the transverse process (arrows) in relation to the body of the superior vertebra. **(C)** Lateral radiograph of the same specimen. Barium paste was applied to the transverse process to outline its image (arrows). Depending on the angle of the x-ray tube or the position of the patient, any portion of the transverse process may superimpose the vertebral body to produce a Mach band similar to that seen in **A**. *Source*: Reprinted with permission from ''Pseudofractures of the Cervical Vertebral Body'' by RH Daffner, ZL Deeb, and WE Rothfus in *Skeletal Radiology* (1986;15:295–298), Copyright © 1986, Springer-Verlag.

C

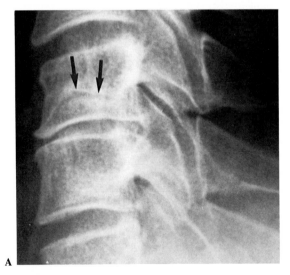

A

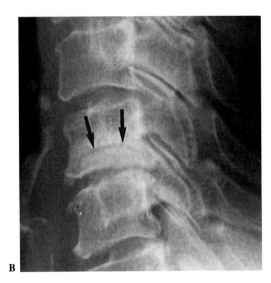

B

Figure 6-15 Mach bands of the vertebral body due to uncinate spurring. **(A and B)** Two different patients with degenerative changes in the vertebral column show curvilinear lucencies through the bodies of C-5 (arrows). This is a common phenomenon in older individuals with cervical spondylosis and occurs most often at C-5, C-6, and C-7.

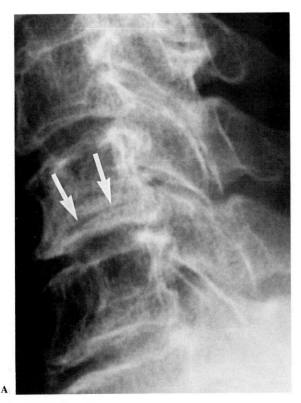 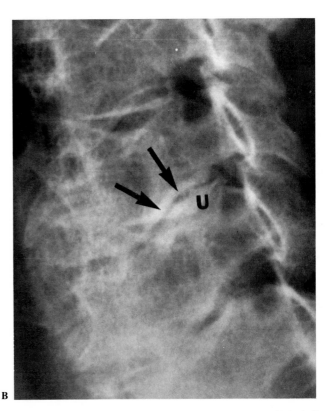

Figure 6-16 Pseudofracture (Mach bands) due to an osteophyte. **(A)** Lateral radiograph shows a curvilinear lucency along the base of C-5 (arrows). This is similar to those demonstrated in Fig 6-15. **(B)** Oblique radiograph shows that the lucency is due to overlap of a prominent osteophyte of the vertebral body (arrows) in close proximity to osteophytes of the uncinate process (U).

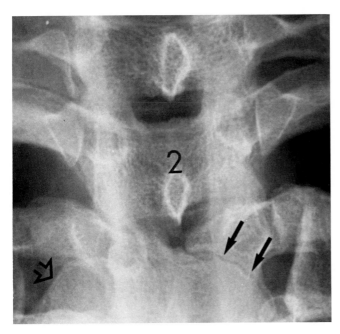

Figure 6-17 Mach band due to sternal interposition. There is a curvilinear lucency across the left side of the body of T-3 (long arrows). This is due to the overlap of the manubrium sterni over T-3. The margin of the right side of the manubrium (open arrow) does not overlap the vertebra.

Subjective Contours

Subjective contours are a curious psychophysiologic phenomenon in which a geometric figure is constructed psychologically by integrating information from partial lines (Figs 6-18 and 6-19). Under normal circumstances, contours are perceived because of sudden changes in the brightness or color of adjacent areas that stimulate the retina. The phenomenon works for curvilinear structures as well as for straight lines. The term subjective contours is used because the outlines are perceived but are not real. They exist as a real presence only in the observer's visual experience.

Subjective contour images have certain characteristics in common. First, the area contained by a subjective contour appears to be more prominent or even brighter than the background (Fig 6-18). This most likely is the result of lateral inhibition similar to that occurring in Mach band formation. Second, the region subtended by the contours appears to be superimposed over adjacent structures (Fig 6-19). Third, subjective contours may be generated in the absence of straight lines. Because geometric regularity is not a prerequisite for contour formation, this greatly influences the perception of

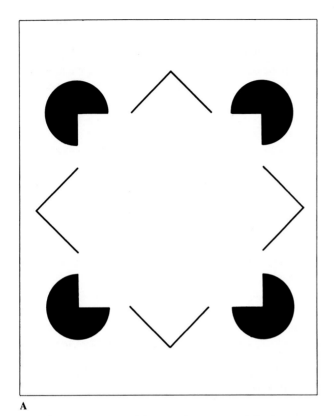

A

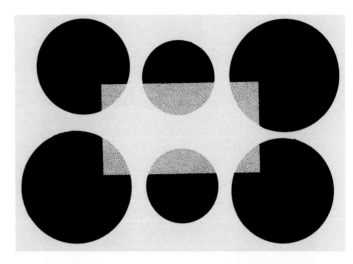

Figure 6-19 Subjective contours. The shaded areas of each circle give rise to the image of a transparent rectangle superimposed on those circles. *Source*: Reprinted from *Applied Radiology* (1984;13[4]:96–98) with the permission of Brentwood Publishing Corporation, a Prentice-Hall/Simon & Schuster unit of Gulf + Westsern Inc.

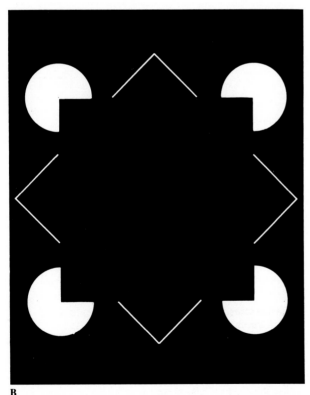

B

Figure 6-18 Subjective contours. A rectangle appears to be superimposed on another rectangle as well as on the circles. The effect occurs even when the images are reversed. Furthermore, in **A**, the center white rectangle appears to be whiter than the background; in **B**, the center black rectangle appears to be blacker than the background. *Source*: Reprinted from *Applied Radiology* (1984;13[4]:96–98) with the permission of Brentwood Publishing Corporation, a Prentice-Hall/Simon & Schuster unit of Gulf + Western Inc.

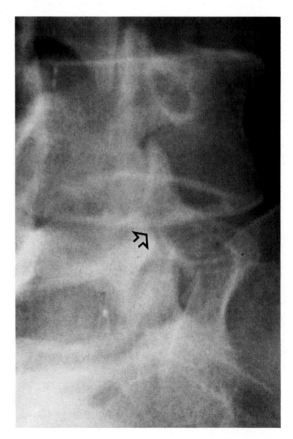

Figure 6-20 Pseudopars defect of L-5. There is an oblique lucency across the pars (open arrow) due to the close proximity of a sclerotic pars and the pedicle shadow. Tomograms showed no evidence of fracture.

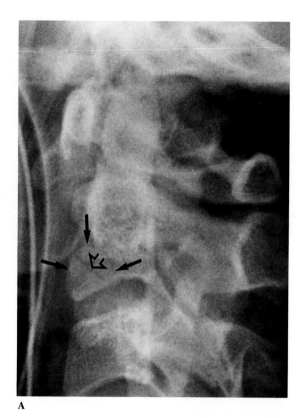

A

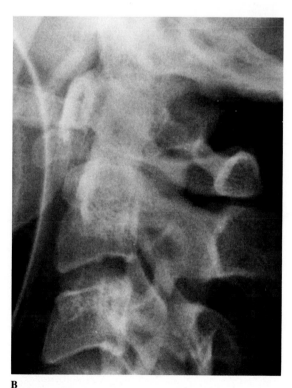

B

Figure 6-21 Pseudofracture due to a plastic rivet on a restraining collar. **(A)** Lateral radiograph shows an oblique lucency across the base of C-2 (open arrow). On careful inspection, there is a curvilinear density containing this lucency (solid arrows). **(B)** The lucency is no longer present after removal of the collar. *Source*: Reprinted with permission from "Pseudofractures due to Nec-Loc Cervical Immobilization Collar" by RH Daffner and MB Khoury in *Skeletal Radiology* (1987;16:460–462), Copyright © 1987, Springer-Verlag.

false outlines on a radiograph. Finally, close examination of subjective contours makes them disappear because they have no physical basis. Magnifying the area in question will also result in the disappearance of the contour. If the entire area is viewed without magnification, the contour will reappear.

From a clinical standpoint, the one area in the vertebral column where subjective contour formation is most likely to occur is on oblique radiographs of the lumbar region. In this situation, the close proximity of a sclerotic pars interarticularis and the normally sclerotic line of the adjacent pedicle result in the false perception of a lucency across the pars (Fig 6-20). In this region, subjective contour formation is enhanced by the presence of background contrast effect, another psycho-physiologic phenomenon related to Mach band formation in which differences in background density affect the perception of adjacent structures. Tomography or additional views may be required to clear the area in question.

Occasionally, lucencies due to the rivets of a restraining neck collar may overlie a vertebra.[4] This is a common finding and may be resolved by the removal of the cervical collar (Fig 6-21). Technically, this is a variant of subjective contour formation.

Table 6-1 summarizes the common pseudofractures of the vertebral column.

Table 6-1 Common Vertebral Pseudofractures

Mach Bands

1. Base of dens, frontal view
2. Posterior arches, oblique view
3. Uncinate process on disk, lateral view
4. Uncinate spurs, lateral view
5. Transverse process, lateral view
6. Osteophytes, lateral view
7. Sternum, frontal view

Subjective Contours

1. Pars interarticularis, oblique views
2. Collar rivets

Variants

1. Failure of fusion
2. Cleft sulcus of vertebral artery of atlas
3. Differential growth rates of C-1 and C-2 in children
4. Spurlike deformities in lateral masses of C-1
5. Os odontoideum
6. Ossification of center of tip of dens
7. Synchondrosis of base of dens
8. Cleft body of C-2
9. Ununited ring apophysis
10. Cervical pseudosubluxation in children
11. Intercalary bones
12. Ossification of ligamentum nuchae
13. Scheuermann's disease
14. Vertebral edge separation (Schmorl's variant)

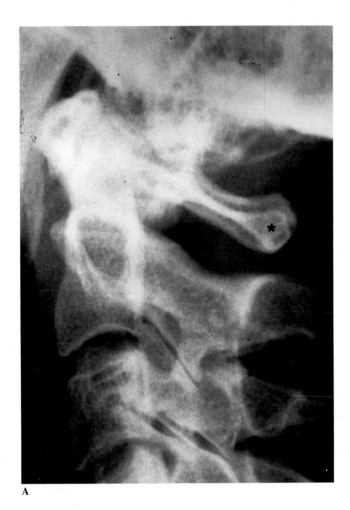

A

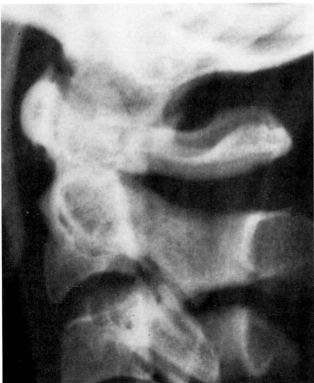

B

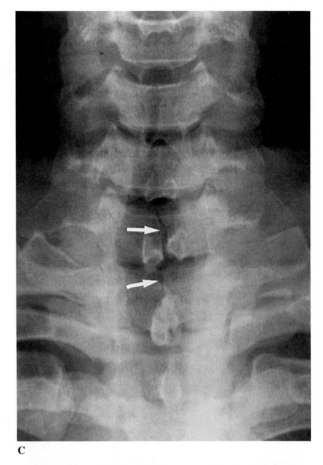

C

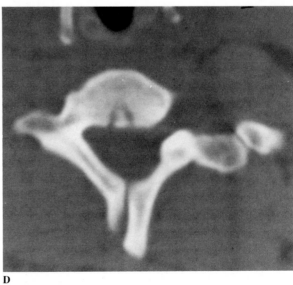

D

Figure 6-22 Spinal dysraphism. **(A)** Failure of fusion of the posterior arch of C-1. Lateral radiograph shows absence of the arch canal line in C-1 (∗). **(B)** Another patient with a similar finding. Occasionally these clefts may be superimposed on the anterior arch of C-1 or the dens and may be misinterpreted as a fracture on the frontal view. **(C)** Failure of fusion of the spinous processes of C-7 and T-1 (arrows), producing vertical lucencies in the two vertebrae. **(D)** CT scan of the same patient shows the well-defined cleft posteriorly.

NORMAL VARIANTS

There are literally hundreds of variants that may occur within the vertebral column. Keats, in his *Atlas of Normal Roentgen Variants That May Simulate Disease*,[13] devotes more than 100 pages and shows more than 200 examples of various anomalies. Many of these may be confused with fractures or dislocations. Since a complete catalog of such anomalies is beyond the scope of this book, this portion of the chapter describes and illustrates some of the variants that are not only more common but also are most likely to cause diagnostic difficulty when encountered in a patient who has suffered vertebral trauma.

Cervical Column

Most of the variants encountered in the cervical column occur at C-1 and C-2. Anomalies of the atlas vertebra occur more often than other anomalies. The most common of these variants is failure of fusion of the posterior arch of the atlas.[8] This may be easily recognized on the lateral radiograph by the absence of the spinolaminar line at C-1 (Fig 6-22). Although this anomaly is rarely a cause for concern, the failure of fusion when viewed on an oblique view could be misinterpreted as a fracture of the posterior arch.

Other arch anomalies may range from simple failure of fusion of one of the rings of the atlas to complete agenesis (Fig 6-23). Arch anomalies of the atlas may, however, be associated with unilateral or bilateral lateral atlanto-axial offset of up to 2 mm (Fig 6-24). These must be differentiated from the offset encountered with a burst fracture of Jefferson. As a rule, Jefferson fractures have lateral atlanto-axial offset greater than 3 mm (Fig 6-25).[8]

Another arch anomaly of the atlas is a cleft through the sulcus of the vertebral artery (Fig 6-26). Careful inspection of the defect will show a sclerotic margin around the cleft. Such clefts are often bilateral.[8]

Differential growth between the atlas and axis in young children often results in bilateral lateral atlanto-axial offset (Fig 6-27). The degree of offset may be quite striking. This is a normal physiologic variant and not a Jefferson fracture (which is unusual in young children).[10]

Linear spurlike deformities of the medial aspect of the lateral masses of the atlas are normal variants that should not be mistaken for lateral mass fractures. These are often bilateral and symmetrical (Fig 6-28).[11,13]

The normal ossification center of the tip of the dens usually appears at age 2 and fuses by age 12 (Fig 6-29). This should not be mistaken for a fracture of the tip of the dens. The so-called type 1 dens fracture, which involves the tip of the dens

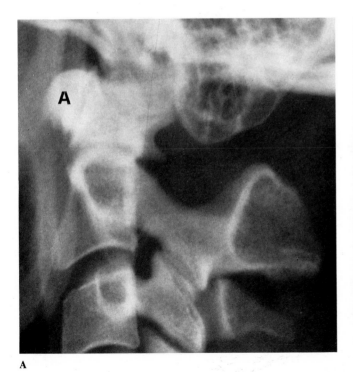
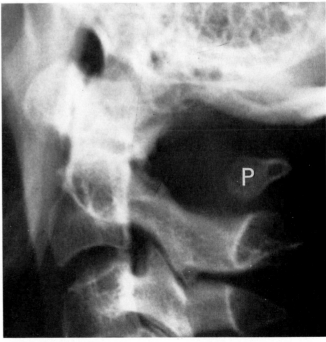

A   B

Figure 6-23 Arch anomalies of C-1. Both these cases were associated with bilateral lateral atlanto-axial offset. **(A)** Complete absence of the posterior arch of C-1. The anterior arch (A) is present. **(B)** Partial absence of the posterior arches of C-1. The lateral view shows the posterior-most portion of the posterior arch (P). The remainder of the posterior arch is absent. *Source:* Reprinted with permission from ''Malformations of the Atlas Vertebra Simulating the Jefferson Fracture'' by JA Gehweiler Jr, RH Daffner, and L Roberts Jr in *American Journal of Roentgenology* (1983;140:1083–1086), Copyright © 1983, American Roentgen Ray Society.

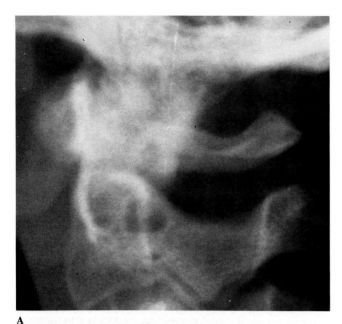

A

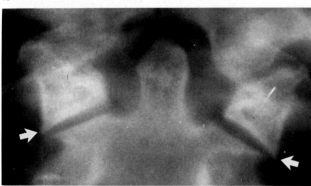

B

Figure 6-24 Bilateral lateral atlanto-axial offset in a patient in whom the posterior arch of the atlas did not fuse. **(A)** Lateral radiograph shows absence of the arch canal line of C-1. **(B)** Frontal tomograms show the bilateral lateral atlanto-axial offset (arrows). *Source*: Reprinted with permission from ''Malformations of the Atlas Vertebra Simulating the Jefferson Fracture'' by JA Gehweiler Jr, RH Daffner, and L Roberts Jr in *American Journal of Roentgenology* (1983;140:1083–1086), Copyright © 1983, American Roentgen Ray Society.

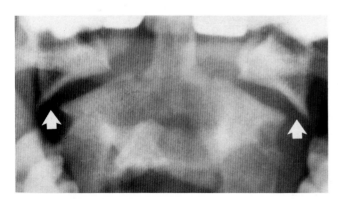

Figure 6-25 Jefferson fracture. An altanto-axial view shows bilateral lateral atlanto-axial offset. In this instance, the degree of offset is greater than 3 mm bilaterally. Note the widening of the space between the dens and the lateral masses. A CT scan confirmed the Jefferson fracture.

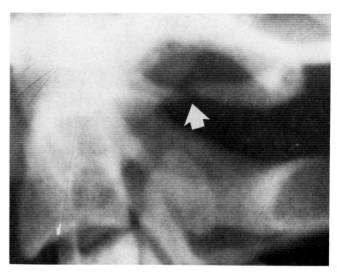

Figure 6-26 Cleft in C-1 through the sulcus of the vertebral artery (arrow). This is another anomaly associated with bilateral lateral atlanto-axial offset. *Source*: Reprinted with permission from ''Malformations of the Atlas Vertebra Simulating the Jefferson Fracture'' by JA Gehweiler Jr, RH Daffner, and L Roberts Jr in *American Journal of Roentgenology* (1983;140:1083–1086), Copyright © 1983, American Roentgen Ray Society.

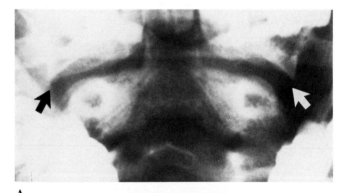

A

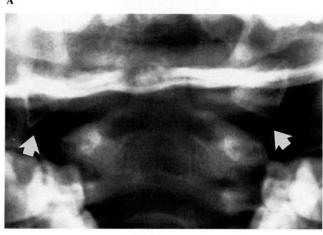

B

Figure 6-27 (A and B) Bilateral lateral atlanto-axial offset (arrows) in two different children due to the disparity of growth rates between C-1 and C-2. The offset was great enough in **B** to require a CT scan to confirm that there was no evidence of Jefferson fracture.

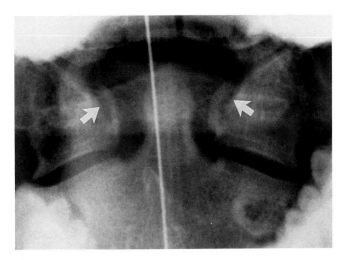

Figure 6-28 Vertical clefts of the lateral masses of C-1 (arrows).

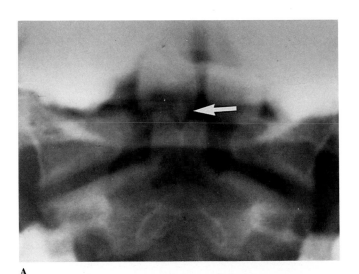

A

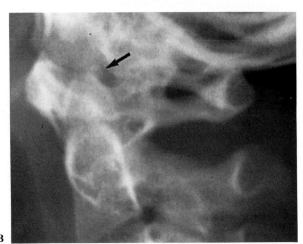

B

Figure 6-29 Normal ossification center of the tip of the dens in a child. **(A)** Atlanto-axial view shows a small terminal ossicle (arrow). **(B)** The lateral radiograph shows that the ossicle is located posteriorly (arrow). There is evidence to suggest that the so-called type I dens fractures are congenital anomalies. *Source*: Courtesy of Dr T Keats, Charlottesville, VA.

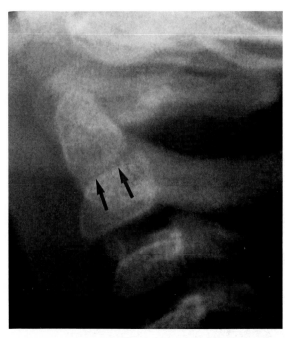

Figure 6-30 Normal synchondrosis of the base of the dens in a young child (arrows). This common anomaly should never be misinterpreted as a fracture. *Source*: Courtesy of Dr E Effman, Durham, NC.

and is considered rare, is probably an unfused apophysis rather than a fracture.[11,13]

In young children, the synchondrosis of the base of the dens may appear as a lucency across the base of that structure. Quite often, sclerotic margins may be seen in conjunction with this abnormality (Fig 6-30). Harris' ring is intact.[13] There are normally clefts at the base of the dens that develop in a vertical or V-shaped fashion. These, too, are remnants of a synchondrosis and should not be mistaken for a fracture, particularly when they are unilateral (Fig 6-31).[12,13]

Failure of union of the dens may result in a separate os odontoideum (Fig 6-32). In this anomaly, the bony margin of the os odontoideum and the body of C-2 are smooth and rounded. There may be overgrowth of the anterior arch of the atlas to compensate.[6,7,11,13]

Ununited ring apophyses (Fig 6-33) may be misinterpreted as a fracture. These usually occur along the superior and inferior surfaces of the anterior aspect of the vertebral bodies in young children. They are extremely common.[11,13]

The cervical vertebral column in children is quite mobile. With even minor degrees of flexion, pseudosubluxation may occur (Fig 6-34).[10] The spinolaminar line is important in establishing whether a true subluxation has occurred. In pseudosubluxation, the spinolaminar line appears to be intact. A similar phenomenon may be encountered in patients with degenerative disk disease (Fig 6-35). In these instances loss of disk height may result in anterolisthesis or retrolisthesis of the body of the vertebra, but the spinolaminar line remains relatively intact.

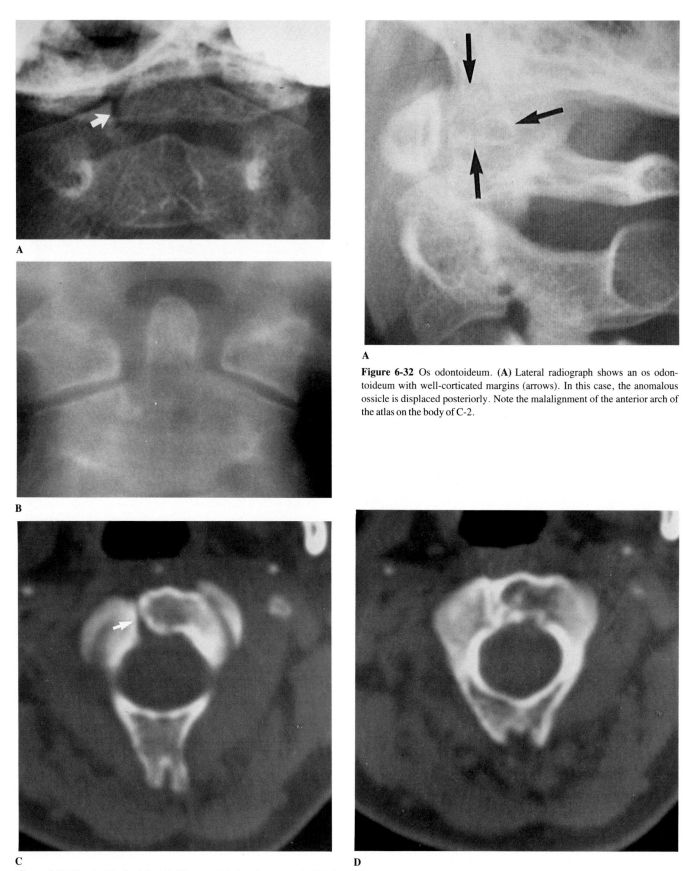

A

B

A

Figure 6-32 Os odontoideum. **(A)** Lateral radiograph shows an os odontoideum with well-corticated margins (arrows). In this case, the anomalous ossicle is displaced posteriorly. Note the malalignment of the anterior arch of the atlas on the body of C-2.

C

D

Figure 6-31 Vertebral body cleft. **(A)** Altanto-axial view shows a vertical V-shaped lucency on the right side of the vertebral body adjacent to the dens (arrow). In most instances, these clefts are bilateral (see Figs 6-5, 6-6A, 6-8B, 6-25, and 6-28). **(B)** Frontal tomogram through this area shows no evidence of fracture. **(C)** CT scan through the area of the cleft shows the lucency (arrow). **(D)** The CT section slightly lower shows no evidence of fracture.

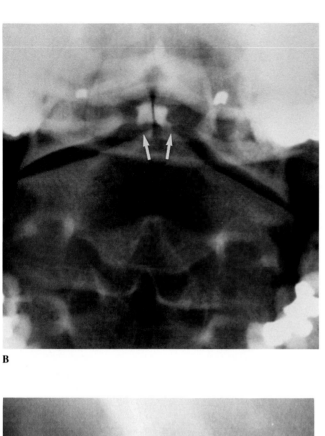

B

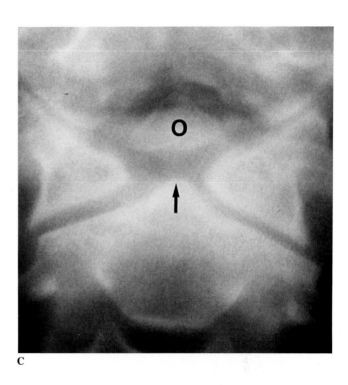

C

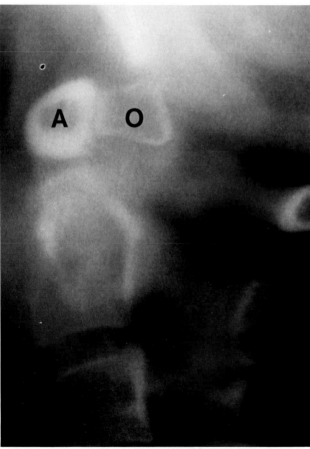

D

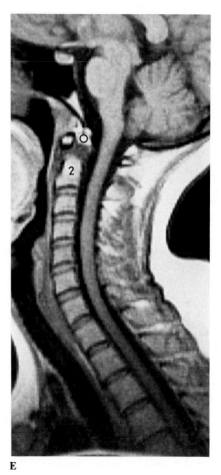

E

Figure 6-32 (B) Atlanto-axial view shows the rounded margin of the base of the dens (arrows). **(C)** Frontal tomogram shows the rounded margin of the base of the dens (arrow) and the free ununited ossicle (O). **(D)** Lateral tomogram shows the relationships in detail. There is nearly complete fusion between the ossicle (O) and the anterior arch of the atlas (A). **(E)** Sagittal MRI study ($T_R = 0.3$, $T_E = 35$) shows the relationship of the ossicle (O) to the body of C-2. There is no evidence of encroachment on the spinal cord.

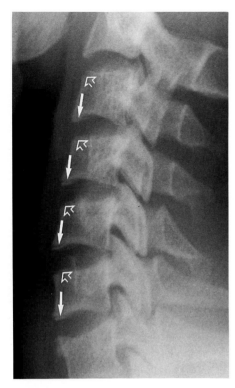

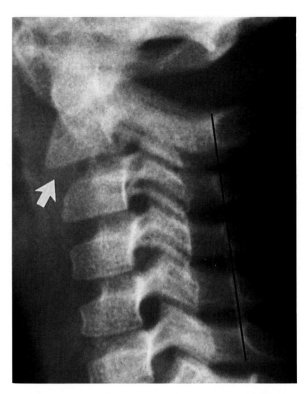

Figure 6-33 Normal ring apophyses of the cervical vertebral column in a teen-age boy. The apophyses occur superiorly (open arrows) as well as inferiorly (solid arrows).

Figure 6-34 Pseudosubluxation of C-2 on C-3 in a young child. The anterior portion of the body of C-2 appears to be displaced over C-3 (arrow). The spinolaminar line (drawn in) is normal.

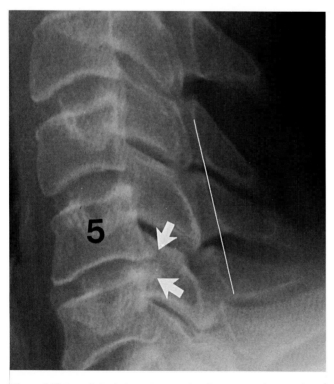

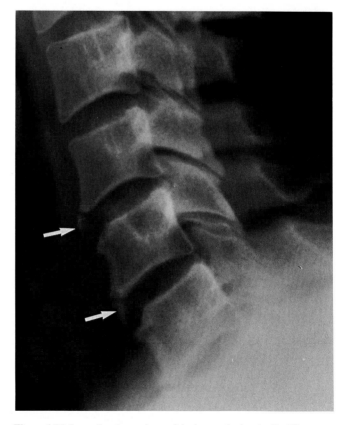

Figure 6-35 Retrolisthesis due to degenerative disease. Posterior osteophytes at the C-5 disk level (arrows) are encroaching on the vertebral canal. There is narrowing of the C-5 disk space and slight posterior displacement of the spinolaminar line (drawn in) above C-6.

Figure 6-36 Intercalary bones (arrows) in the anterior longitudinal ligament.

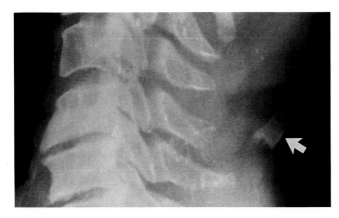

Figure 6-37 Ossification of the ligamentum nuchae (arrow). This should not be misinterpreted as a spinous process fracture.

Finally, intercalary bones within the anterior longitudinal ligament at the level of the intervertebral disk space should not be misinterpreted as a fracture (Fig 6-36). These structures occur quite commonly in older patients. Similarly, ossification in the ligamentum nuchae (Fig 6-37) should not be misinterpreted as a fracture of a spinous process.

These variants and others are illustrated in Keats' atlas.[13]

Thoracic Column

The variants in the thoracic column that are most likely to result in a misdiagnosis of a fracture are ununited ring apophyses and Scheuermann's disease.[13] Ununited ring apophyses cause a curling on the superior, anteroinferior aspects of the vertebral bodies (Fig 6-38). They frequently have sclerotic margins and occur in young individuals. These findings should be sufficient to allow a proper diagnosis to be made. In Scheuermann's disease, osteochondrosis of ring apophyses may result in irregularity and perhaps in fragmentation of the ring apophyses (Fig 6-39).[13] Tomography may be necessary to establish the correct diagnosis by showing extensive involvement along the disk margin.

Lumbar Column

As in the thoracic column, ununited ring apophyses may be misinterpreted as fractures of the edges of vertebral bodies (Fig 6-40). These abnormalities often look quite similar to the vertebral edge separation (limbus vertebra), which occurs as a result of herniation of disk material through the vertebral body (Figs 6-41 and 6-42). As such, they are related to Schmorl's node (Fig 6-43). Smooth sclerotic borders are the key to the differential diagnosis of these abnormalities from simple compression fractures (Fig 6-44). Occasionally, a vertebral edge separation may occur along the posterior surface of the vertebral body (Fig 6-45).

These variants and additional, less common ones are also illustrated in Keats' atlas.[13]

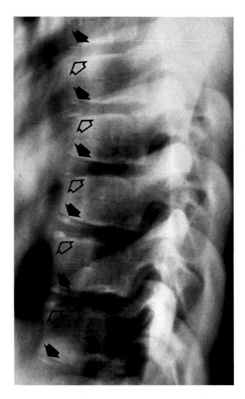

Figure 6-38 Ununited ring apophyses superiorly (open arrows) and inferiorly (solid arrows) in a teen-age boy.

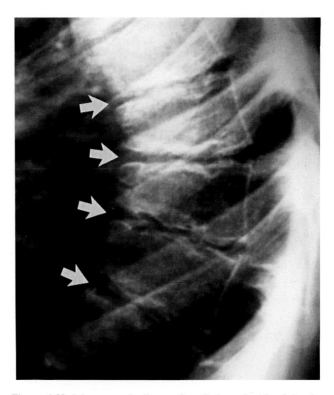

Figure 6-39 Scheuermann's disease. So-called apophysitis of the ring apophyses has caused anterior wedging of several vertebral bodies and irregularity along the disk margins (arrows). Kyphotic deformity has occurred as a result.

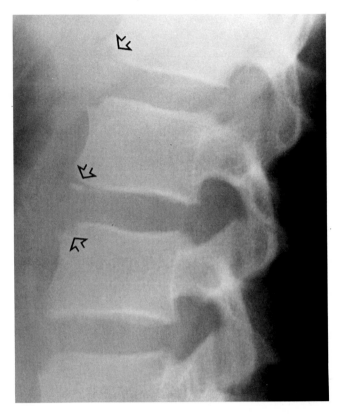

Figure 6-40 Normal ring apophyses (arrows) in the lumbar region of a teenager.

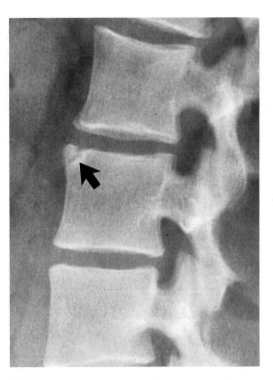

Figure 6-41 Vertebral edge separation ("limbus vertebra") (arrow). This occurs as a result of anterior herniation of disk material through the anterosuperior lip of the vertebral body. There is a sclerotic margin along the border of the body. The vertebral disk space above the abnormal vertebra is usually narrowed.

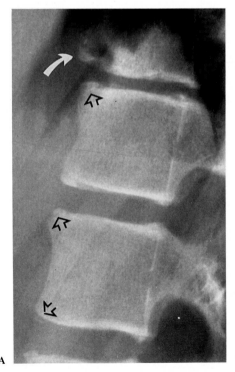

A

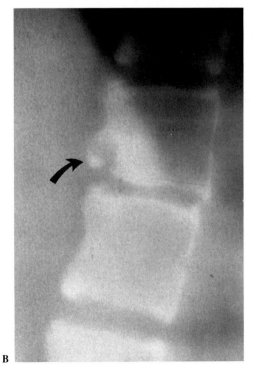

B

Figure 6-42 Inferior vertebral edge separation in a young individual. (A) Lateral radiograph shows a small separated fragment of bone (curved arrow). Note the normal ring apophyses (open arrows). (B) Lateral tomogram shows the free bony fragment (arrow). Note the sclerotic margin (diskogenic sclerosis) in the underlying vertebra.

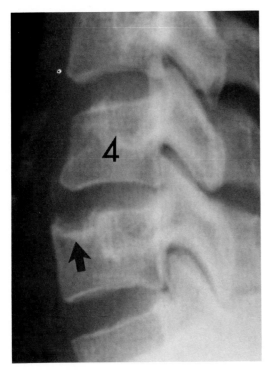

Figure 6-43 Cervical Schmorl's node (arrow). This abnormality is caused by intraosseous herniation of disk material. The lesion has a sclerotic margin. Schmorl's nodes are most commonly found in the thoracic and lumbar vertebrae. There often is associated diskogenic sclerosis of the vertebral body adjacent to the lesion.

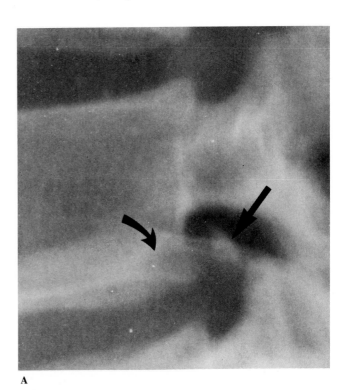

A

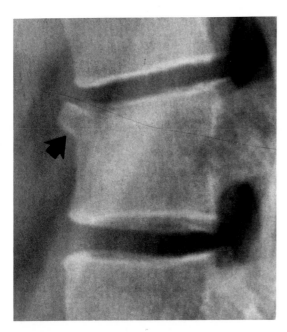

Figure 6-44 Simple compression fracture of L-1 (arrow). Simple compression fractures can easily be differentiated from vertebral edge separation due to disk herniation. In the former condition, the bone fragment can (mentally) be put back into place like a jigsaw puzzle piece. In the latter instance, the pieces will not fit snugly. Both conditions are often accompanied by narrowing of the disk space above the lesion. Compare with Figs 6-41 and 6-42.

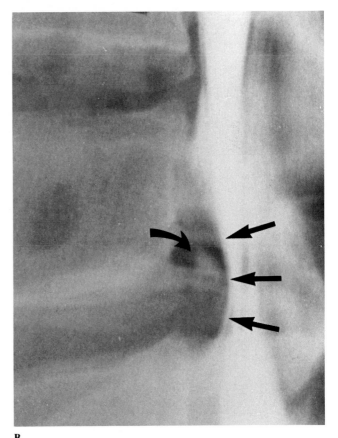

B

Figure 6-45 Posterior vertebral edge separation. **(A)** Lateral radiograph shows a fragment of bone within the vertebral canal (straight arrow). The bony defect that has resulted from this rarest of vertebral edge separations due to disk disease is also visible (curved arrow). **(B)** Lateral myelogram shows an extradural defect compressing the thecal sac (straight arrows). The bone fragment (curved arrow) is again seen.

REFERENCES

1. Daffner RH: Visual illusions affecting perception of the roentgen image. *CRC Crit Rev Diagn Imaging* 1983;20:79–119.

2. Daffner RH: Pseudofracture of the dens: Mach bands. *AJR* 1977;128:607–612.

3. Daffner RH, Gehweiler JA Jr: Pseudovacuum of the cervical intervertebral disc: A normal variant. *AJR* 1981;137:737–739.

4. Daffner RH, Khoury MB: Pseudofractures due to Nec-Loc cervical immobilization collar. *Skeletal Radiol* 1987;16:460–462.

5. Daffner RH, Deeb ZL, Rothfus WE: Pseudofractures of the cervical vertebral body. *Skeletal Radiol* 1986;15:295–298.

6. Fielding JW, Griffin PP: Os odontoideum: An acquired lesion. *J Bone Joint Surg* 1974;56A:187–190.

7. Fielding JW, Hensinger RN, Hawkins RJ: Os odontoideum. *J Bone Joint Surg* 1980;62A:376–383.

8. Gehweiler JA Jr, Daffner RH, Roberts L Jr: Malformations of the atlas vertebra simulating the Jefferson fracture. *AJR* 1983;140:1083–1086.

9. Goldberg RP, Vine HS, Sacks BA, et al: The cervical split: A pseudofracture. *Skeletal Radiol* 1982;7:267–272.

10. Jacobson G, Bleecker HH: Pseudosubluxation of the axis in children. *AJR* 1959;82:472–481.

11. Kattan KR: *"Trauma" and "No-Trauma" of the Cervical Spine.* Springfield, Ill, Charles C Thomas Publisher, 1975.

12. Kattan KR: Two features of the atlas vertebra simulating fractures by tomography. *AJR* 1979;132:963–965.

13. Keats TE: *Atlas of Normal Roentgen Variants That May Simulate Disease*, ed 3. Chicago, Year Book Medical Publishers, 1984, pp 157–263.

General References

Abel MS: *Occult Traumatic Lesions of the Cervical Vertebrae*. St Louis, Warren H Green Inc, 1971.

Abel MS: Occult traumatic lesions of the cervical spine. *CRC Crit Rev Clin Radiol Nucl Med* 1975;7:469–553.

Abel MS: The exaggerated supine oblique view of the cervical spine. *Skeletal Radiol* 1982;8:213–219.

Acheson MB, Livingston RR, Richardson ML, et al: High-resolution CT scanning in the evaluation of cervical spine fractures: Comparison with plain film examinations. *AJR* 1987;148:1179–1185.

Alker GJ Jr, Oh YS, Leslie EV, et al: Postmortem radiology of head and neck injuries in fatal traffic accidents. *Radiology* 1975;114:611–617.

Amyes EW, Anderson FM: Fracture of the odontoid process: Report of sixty-three cases. *Arch Surg* 1956;72:377–393.

Anderson JE: *Grant's Atlas of Anatomy,* ed 8. Baltimore, Williams & Wilkins, 1983, pp 5-1–5-23.

Anderson LD, D'Alonzo RT: Fractures of the odontoid process of the axis. *J Bone Joint Surg* 1974;56A:1663–1674.

Atlas SW, Regenbogen V, Rogers LF, et al: The radiographic characterization of burst fractures of the spine. *AJR* 1986;147:575–582.

Banna M: *Clinical Radiology of the Spine and the Spinal Cord*. Rockville, MD, Aspen Publishers, Inc, 1985, pp 1–158.

Binet EF, Moro JJ, Marangola JP, et al: Cervical spine tomography in trauma. *Spine* 1977;2:163–172.

Blockey NJ, Purser DW: Fractures of the odontoid process of the axis. *J Bone Joint Surg* 1956;38B:794–817.

Bohlman HH: Acute fractures and dislocations of the cervical spine—an analysis of three hundred hospitalized patients and review of the literature. *J Bone Joint Surg* 1979;61:1119–1142.

Braakman R, Penning L: *Injuries of the Cervical Spine*. London, Excerpta Medica, 1971.

Braakman R, Vinken PJ: Unilateral facet interlocking in the lower cervical spine. *J Bone Joint Surg* 1967;49B:249–257.

Brant-Zawadzki M, Jeffrey RB, Minagi H, et al: High resolution CT of thoracolumbar fractures. *AJNR* 1982;3:69–74.

Brant-Zawadzki M, Miller EM, Federle MP: CT in the evaluation of spine trauma. *AJR* 1981;136:369–375.

Breasted JH: *The Edwin Smith Surgical Papyrus*. Chicago, University of Chicago Press, 1930.

Burke DC: Hyperextension injuries of the spine. *J Bone Joint Surg* 1971;53B:3–12.

Calenoff L, Chessare JW, Rogers LF, et al: Multiple level spinal injuries: Importance of early recognition. *AJR* 1978;130:665–669.

Cancelmo JJ Jr: Clay shoveler's fracture: A helpful diagnostic sign. *AJR* 1972;115:540–543.

Cattell HS, Filtzer DL: Pseudosubluxation and other normal variations of the cervical spine in children: A study of one hundred and sixty children. *J Bone Joint Surg* 1965; 47A:1295–1309.

Chakeres DW, Flickinger F, Bresnahan JC, et al: MR imaging of acute spinal cord trauma. *AJNR* 1987;8:5–10.

Chance GQ: Note on a type of flexion fracture of the spine. *Br J Radiol* 1948;21:452–453.

Charlton OP, Gehweiler JA Jr, Morgan CL, et al: Spondylolysis and spondylolisthesis of the cervical spine. *Skeletal Radiol* 1978;3:79–84.

Cintron E, Gilula LA, Murphy WA, et al: The widened disk space: A sign of cervical hyperextension injury. *Radiology* 1981;141:639–644.

Clark WM, Gehweiler JA, Laib R: Twelve significant signs of cervical spine trauma. *Skeletal Radiol* 1979;3:201–205.

Cohen WA, Young W, DeCrescito V, et al: Posttraumatic syrinx formation: Experimental study. *AJNR* 1985; 6:823–827.

Daffner RH, Deeb ZL, Rothfus WE: "Fingerprints" of vertebral trauma—A unifying concept based on mechanisms. *Skeletal Radiol* 1986;15:518–525.

Daffner RH, Lupetin AR, Dash N, et al: MRI in the detection of malignant infiltration of bone marrow. *AJR* 1986; 146:353–358.

Daffner RH, Deeb ZL, Rothfus WE: The posterior vertebral body line: Importance in the detection of burst fractures. *AJR* 1987;148:93–96.

Daffner RH, Khoury MB: Pseudofractures due to Nec-Loc cervical immobilization collar. *Skeletal Radiol* 1987; 16:460–462.

Daffner RH, Deeb ZL, Rothfus WE: Pseudofractures of the cervical vertebral body. *Skeletal Radiol* 1986;15:295–298.

Daffner RH: Pseudofracture of the dens: Mach bands. *AJR* 1977;128:607–612.

Daffner RH, Gehweiler JA Jr: Pseudovacuum of the cervical intervertebral disc: A normal variant. *AJR* 1981; 137:737–739.

Daffner RH, Deeb ZL, Rothfus WE: Thoracic fractures and dislocations in motorcyclists. *Skeletal Radiol* 1987; 16:280–284.

Daffner RH: Visual illusions affecting perception of the roentgen image. *CRC Crit Rev Diagn Imaging* 1983;20:79–119.

Daffner RH: Injuries of the thoracolumbar vertebral column, in Dalinka MK and Kaye JJ (eds): *Radiology in Emergency Medicine*. New York, Churchill Livingstone, 1984, pp 317–341.

Dehner JR: Seatbelt injuries of the spine and abdomen. *AJR* 1971;111:833–843.

Denis F: The three column spine and its significance in the classification of acute thoracolumbar spinal injuries. *Spine* 1983;8:817–831.

Denis F: Spinal instability as defined by the three-column spine concept in acute spinal trauma. *Clin Orthop* 1984; 189:65–76.

Dolan KD: Cervical spine injuries below the axis. *Radiol Clin North Am* 1977;15:247–259.

Dolan KD: Cervicobasilar relationships. *Radiol Clin North Am* 1977;15:155–166.

Edeiken-Monroe B, Wagner LK, Harris JH Jr: Hyperextension dislocation of the cervical spine. *AJR* 1986;146: 803–808.

Elliott JM Jr, Rogers LF, Wessinger JP, et al: The hangman's fracture. *Radiology* 1972;104:303–307.

England AC, Shippel AH, Ray MJ: A simple view for demonstration of fractures of the anterior arch of C1. *AJR* 1985; 144:763–764.

Epstein BS: *The Spine: A Radiologic Text and Atlas,* ed 4. Philadelphia, Lea & Febiger, 1976.

Ferguson RL, Allen BL Jr: A mechanistic classification of thoracolumbar spine fractures. *Clin Orthop* 1984; 189:77–88.

Fielding JW, Griffin PP: Os odontoideum: An acquired lesion. *J Bone Joint Surg* 1974;56A:187–190.

Fielding JW, Hawkins RJ: Atlanto-axial rotatory fixation: Fixed rotatory subluxation of the atlanto-axial joint. *J Bone Joint Surg* 1977;59A:37–44.

Fielding JW, Hensinger RN, Hawkins RJ: Os odontoideum. *J Bone Joint Surg* 1980;62A:376–383.

Fielding JW, Stillwell WT, Chynn KY, et al: Use of computed tomography for the diagnosis of atlanto-axial rotatory fixation. *J Bone Joint Surg* 1978;60A:1102–1104.

Forsyth HF: Extension injuries of the cervical spine. *J Bone Joint Surg* 1964;46A:1792–1797.

Gehweiler JA Jr, Clark WM, Schaaf RE, et al: Cervical spine trauma: The common combined conditions. *Radiology* 1979;130:77–86.

Gehweiler JA Jr, Daffner RH, Osborne RL Jr: Relevant signs of stable and unstable thoracolumbar vertebral column trauma. *Skeletal Radiol* 1981;7:179–183.

Gehweiler JA Jr, Daffner RH, Roberts L Jr: Malformations of the atlas vertebra simulating the Jefferson fracture. *AJNR* 1983;4:187–190.

Gehweiler JA Jr, Duff DE, Martinez S, et al: Fractures of the atlas vertebra. *Skeletal Radiol* 1976;1:97–102.

Gehweiler JA Jr, Osborne RL Jr, Becker RF: *The Radiology of Vertebral Trauma*. Philadelphia, WB Saunders, 1980.

Gellad FE, Levine AM, Joslyn JN, et al: Pure thoracolumbar facet dislocation: Clinical features and CT appearance. *Radiology* 1986;161:505–508.

Gelman MI, Umber JS: Fractures of the thoracolumbar spine in ankylosing spondylitis. *AJR* 1978;130:485–491.

Goldberg RP, Vine HS, Sacks BA, et al: The cervical split: A pseudofracture. *Skeletal Radiol* 1982;7:267–272.

Goss CM: *Gray's Anatomy of the Human Body.* American ed 29. Philadelphia, Lea & Febiger, 1973, pp 100–121, 294–305.

Green JD, Harle TS, Harris JH Jr: Anterior subluxation of the cervical spine: Hyperflexion sprain. *AJNR* 1981; 2:243–350.

Greenberg AD: Atlantoaxial dislocations. *Brain* 1968; 91:655–684.

Grisolia A, Bell RL, Peltier LF: Fractures and dislocations of the spine complicating ankylosing spondylitis. *J Bone Joint Surg* 1967;49A:339–344.

Guerra J Jr, Garfin SR, Resnick D: Vertebral burst fractures: CT analysis of the retropulsed fragment. *Radiology* 1984; 153:769–772.

Hackney DB, Asato R, Joseph PM, et al: Hemorrhage and edema in acute spinal cord compression: Demonstration by MR imaging. *Radiology* 1986;161:387–390.

Handel SF, Lee YY: Computed tomography of spinal fractures. *Radiol Clin North Am* 1981;19:69–89.

Harris JH Jr: Acute injuries of the spine. *Semin Roentgenol* 1978;13:53–68.

Harris JH Jr: Radiographic evaluation of spinal trauma. *Orthop Clin North Am* 1986;17:75–86.

Harris JH Jr, Burke JT, Ray RD, et al: Low (type III) odontoid fracture: A new radiographic sign. *Radiology* 1984; 153:353–356.

Harris JH Jr, Edeiken-Monroe B: *The Radiology of Acute Cervical Spine Trauma,* ed 2. Baltimore, Williams & Wilkins, 1987.

Holdsworth FW: Fractures, dislocations, and fracture-dislocations of the spine. *J Bone Joint Surg* 1963;45B:6–20.

Holdsworth FW: Review article: Fractures, dislocations, and fracture-dislocations of the spine. *J Bone Joint Surg* 1970; 52A:1534–1551.

Jackson H, Kam J, Harris JH Jr, et al: The sacral arcuate lines in upper sacral fractures. *Radiology* 1982;145:35–39.

Jacobson G, Alder DC: An evaluation of lateral atlanto-axial displacement in injuries of the cervical spine. *Radiology* 1953;61:355–362.

Jacobson G, Alder DC: Examination of the atlanto-axial joint following injury with particular emphasis on rotational subluxation. *AJR* 1956;76:1081–1094.

Jacobson G, Bleecker HH: Pseudosubluxation of the axis in children. *AJR* 1959;82:472–481.

Jefferson G: Fracture of the atlas vertebra: Report of four cases, and a review of those previously recorded. *Br J Surg* 1920;7:407–422.

Kattan KR: *"Trauma" and "No-Trauma" of the Cervical Spine.* Springfield, IL, Charles C Thomas Publisher, 1975.

Kattan KR: Two features of the atlas vertebra simulating fractures by tomography. *AJR* 1979;132:963–965.

Kattan KR: Backward "displacement" of the spinolaminar line at C2: A normal variation. *AJR* 1977;129:289–290.

Kattan KR, Pais MJ: Some borderlands of the cervical spine: Part I: The normal (and nearly normal) that may appear pathologic. *Skeletal Radiol* 1982;8:1–6.

Kattan KR, Pais MJ: Some borderlands of the cervical spine: Part II: The subtle and the hidden abnormal. *Skeletal Radiol* 1982;8:7–12.

Kaydoya S, Nakamura T, Kobayashi S, et al: Magnetic resonance imaging of acute spinal cord injury: Report of three cases. *Neuroradiology* 1987;29:252–255.

Keene JS, Goletz TH, Lilleas F, et al: Diagnosis of vertebral fractures: A comparison of conventional radiography, conventional tomography and computed axial tomography. *J Bone Joint Surg* 1982;64A:586–594.

Kilcoyne RF, Mack LA, King HA, et al: Thoracolumbar spine injuries associated with vertical plunges: Reappraisal with computed tomography. *Radiology* 1983;146:137–140.

Kowalski HM, Cohen WA, Cooper P, et al: Pitfalls in the CT diagnosis of atlantoaxial rotary subluxation. *AJNR* 1987; 8:697–702.

Kulkarni MV, McArdle CB, Kopanicky D, et al: *Radiology* 1987;164:837–843.

Lee C, Kim KS, Rogers LF: Triangular cervical vertebral body fractures: Diagnostic significance. *AJR* 1982; 138:1123–1132.

Lee C, Kim KS, Rogers LF: Sagittal fracture of the cervical vertebral body. *AJR* 1982;139:55–60.

Lee C, Rogers LF, Woodring JH, et al: Fractures of the craniovertebral junction associated with other fractures of the spine: Overlooked entity? *AJNR* 1984;5:775–781.

Lee C, Woodring JH, Goldstein SJ, et al: Evaluation of traumatic atlantooccipital dislocations. *AJNR* 1987; 8:19–26.

Lee C, Woodring JH, Rogers LF, et al: The radiographic distinction of degenerative slippage (spondyloslisthesis and retrolisthesis) from traumatic slippage of the cervical spine. *Skeletal Radiol* 1986;15:439–443.

Manaster BJ, Osborn AG: CT patterns of facet fracture dislocations in the thoracolumbar region. *AJNR* 1986; 7:1007–1012.

Maravilla KR, Cooper PR, Sklar FH: The influence of thin-section tomography on the treatment of cervical spine injuries. *Radiology* 1978;128:131–139.

Martinez S, Morgan CL, Gehweiler JA Jr, et al: Unusual fractures and dislocations of the axis vertebra. *Skeletal Radiol* 1979;3:206–212.

Mazur JM, Stauffer ESP: Unrecognized spinal instability associated with seemingly "simple" cervical compression fractures. *Spine* 1983;8:687–692.

McAfee PC, Yuan HA, Lasda NA: The unstable burst fracture. *Spine* 1983;7:365–373.

McArdle CB, Wright JW, Prevost WJ, et al: MR imaging of the acutely injured patient with cervical traction. *Radiology* 1986;159:273–274.

Miller MD, Gehweiler JA Jr, Martinez S, et al: Significant new observations on cervical spine trauma. *AJR* 1978; 130:659–663.

Mirvis SE, Young JWR, Lim C, et al: Hangman's fracture: Radiologic assessment in 27 cases. *Radiology* 1987; 163:713–717.

Montana MA, Richardson ML, Kilcoyne RF, et al: CT of sacral injury. *Radiology* 1986;161:499–503.

Morris RE, Hasso AN, Thompson JR, et al: Traumatic dural tears: CT diagnosis using metrizamide. *Radiology* 1984; 152:443–446.

Naidich JB, Naidich TP, Garfein C, et al: The widened interspinous distance: A useful sign of anterior cervical dislocation in the supine frontal projection. *Radiology* 1977; 123:113–116.

O'Callaghan JP, Ullrich CG, Yuan HA, et al: CT of facet distraction in flexion injuries of the thoracolumbar spine: The "naked" facet. *AJNR* 1980;1:97–102.

Pay NT, George AE, Benjamin MV, et al: Positive and negative contrast myelography in spinal trauma. *Radiology* 1977;123:103–111.

Penning L: Normal movements of the cervical spine. *AJR* 1978;130:317–326.

Penning L: Prevertebral hematoma in cervical spine injury: Incidence and etiologic significance. *AJR* 1981;136: 553–561.

Petras AF, Sobel DF, Mani JR, et al: CT myelography in cervical nerve root avulsion. *J Comput Assist Tomogr* 1985;9(2):275–279.

Post MJD, Green BA: The use of computed tomography in spinal trauma. *Radiol Clin North Am* 1983;21:327–375.

Post MJD, Green BA, Quencer RM, et al: The value of computed tomography in spinal trauma. *Spine* 1982; 7:417–431.

Post MJD, Seminer DS, Quencer RM: CT diagnosis of spinal epidural hematoma. *AJNR* 1982;3:190–192.

Powers B, Miller MD, Kramer RS, et al: Traumatic anterior atlanto-occipital dislocation. *Neurosurgery* 1979;4:12–17.

Reymond RD, Wheeler PS, Perovic M, et al: The lucent cleft, a new radiographic sign of cervical disc injury or disease. *Clin Radiol* 1972;23:188–192.

Roaf R: A study of the mechanics of spinal injuries. *J Bone Joint Surg* 1960;42B:810–823.

Roaf R: International classification of spinal injuries. *Paraplegia* 1972;10:78–84.

Rogers LF: The roentgenographic appearance of transverse or Chance fractures of the spine: The seatbelt fracture. *AJR* 1971;111:844–849.

Rogers LF, Lee C: Cervical spine trauma, in Dalinka MK and Kaye JJ (eds): *Radiology in Emergency Medicine*. New York, Churchill Livingstone, 1984, pp 275–316.

Rogers LF, Thayer C, Weinberg PE, et al: Acute injuries of the upper thoracic spine associated with paraplegia. *AJR* 1980;134:67–73.

Schaaf RE, Gehweiler JA Jr, Powers B, et al: Lateral hyperflexion injuries of the spine. *Skeletal Radiol* 1978;3:73–78.

Schmorl G, Junghanns H: *The Human Spine in Health and Disease*, ed 5. New York, Grune & Stratton, 1971.

Schneider RC, Livingston KE, Cave AJE, et al: "Hangman's fracture" of the cervical spine. *J Neurosurg* 1965;22: 141–154.

Seibert CE, Dreisbach JN, Swanson WB, et al: Progressive posttraumatic cystic myelopathy: Neuroradiologic evaluation. *AJR* 1981;136:1161–1165.

Seljeskog EL, Chous SN: Spectrum of the hangman's fracture. *J Neurosurg* 1976;3:45–48.

Shaffer MA, Doris PE: Limitation of the cross table lateral view in detecting cervical spine injuries: A retrospective analysis. *Ann Emerg Med* 1981;10:508–513.

Shapiro R, Youngberg AS, Rothman SL: The differential diagnosis of traumatic lesions of the occipito-atlanto-axial segment. *Radiol Clin North Am* 1973;11:505–526.

Shargo GG: Cervical spine injuries: Association with head trauma: A review of 50 patients. *AJR* 1973;118:670–673.

Sherk HH, Nicholson JT: Fractures of the atlas. *J Bone Joint Surg* 1970;52A:1017–1024.

Shuman WP, Rogers JV, Sickler ME, et al: Thoracolumbar burst fractures: CT dimensions of the spinal canal relative to postsurgical improvement. *AJNR* 1985;6:337–341.

Smith GR, Abel MS, Cone L: Visualization of the posterolateral elements of the upper cervical vertebrae in the anteroposterior projection. *Radiology* 1975;115:219–220.

Smith GR, Northrop CH, Loop JW: Jumper's fractures: Patterns of thoracolumbar spine injuries associated with vertical plunges. *Radiology* 1977;122:657–663.

Smith WS, Kaufer H: Patterns and mechanisms of lumbar injuries associated with lap seatbelts: *J Bone Joint Surg* 1969;51A:239–254.

Smoker WRK, Dolan KD: The "fat" C2: A sign of fracture. *AJNR* 1987;8:33–38.

Steppé R, Bellemans M, Boven F, et al: The value of computed tomography scanning in elusive fractures of the cervical spine. *Skeletal Radiol* 1981;6:175–178.

Stewart GC, Gehweiler JA Jr, Laib RH, et al: Horizontal fracture of the anterior arch of the atlas. *Radiology* 1977; 122:349–352.

Suss RA, Zimmerman RD, Leeds NE: Pseudospread of the atlas: False sign of Jefferson fracture in young children. *AJNR* 1983;4:183–186.

Swischuk LE: Anterior displacement of C2 in children: Physiologic or pathologic? A helpful differentiating line. *Radiology* 1977;122:759–763.

Tarr RW, Drolshagen LF, Kerner TC, et al: MR imaging of recent spinal trauma. *J Comput Assist Tomogr* 1987; 11:412–417.

Templeton PA, Young JWR, Mirvis SE, et al: The value of retropharyngeal soft tissue measurements in trauma of the adult cervical spine. *Skeletal Radiol* 1987;16:98–104.

Vines FS: The significance of "occult" fractures of the cervical spine. *AJR* 1969;107:493–504.

von Torklus D, Gehle W: *The Upper Cervical Spine: Regional Anatomy, Pathology, and Traumatology: A Systematic Radiological Atlas and Textbook.* New York, Grune & Stratton, 1972.

Whalen JP, Woodruff CL: The cervical prevertebral fat stripe: A new aid in evaluating the cervical prevertebral soft tissue space. *AJR* 1970;109:445–451.

Whitley JE, Forsyth HF: The classification of cervical spine injuries. *AJR* 1960;83:633–644.

Wholey MH, Bruwer AJ, Baker HL: The lateral roentgenogram of the neck (with comments on the atlanto-odontoid basion relationship). *Radiology* 1958;71:350–356.

Wiltse LL, Widell EH, Jackson DW: Fatigue fracture: The basic lesion in isthmic spondylolisthesis. *J Bone Joint Surg* 1975;57A:17–22.

Wojcik WG, Edeiken-Monroe BS, Harris JH Jr: Three-dimensional computed tomography in acute cervical spine trauma: A preliminary report. *Skeletal Radiol* 1987;16:261–269.

Woodring JH, Goldstein SJ: Fractures of the articular processes of the cervical spine. *AJR* 1982;139:341–344.

Woodring JH, Selke AC, Duff DE: Traumatic atlantooccipital dislocation with survival. *AJNR* 1981;2:251–254.

Woodruff FP, Dewing SB: Fracture of the cervical spine in patients with ankylosing spondylitis. *Radiology* 1963; 80:17–21.

Wortzman G, Dewar FP: Rotary fixation of the atlantoaxial joint: Rotational atlantoaxial subluxation. *Radiology* 1968; 90:479–487.

Yetkin Z, Osborn AG, Giles DS, et al: Uncovertebral and facet joint dislocations in cervical articular pillar fractures: CT evaluation. *AJNR* 1985;6:633–637.

Index